HANDBOOK on DRUG and NUTRIENT INTERACTIONS

A reference and study guide

Fifth edition

Daphne A. Roe, MD
PROFESSOR OF NUTRITION
DIVISION OF NUTRITIONAL SCIENCES
CORNELL UNIVERSITY
ITHACA, NY

THE AMERICAN DIETETIC ASSOCIATION

Library of Congress Cataloging-in-Publication Data

Roe, Daphne A., 1923–1993
Handbook on drug and nutrient interactions: a reference and study guide / Daphne A. Roe. — 5th ed.
p. cm.
Includes bibliographical references and indexes.
ISBN 0-88091-135-2
1. Drug-nutrient interactions—Handbooks, manuals, etc.
2. Deficiency diseases—Etiology—Handbooks, manuals, etc.
I. Title
[DNLM: 1. Drug Interactions—handbooks. 2. Nutrition—handbooks.
QV 39 R698h 1994]
RM302.4.R63 1994
615'.7045—dc20
DNLM/DLC
for Library of Congress 94-35993
CIP

The views expressed in this publication are those of the author and do not necessarily reflect policies and/or official positions of The American Dietetic Association. Mention of product names in this publication does not constitute endorsement by the authors or The American Dietetic Association. The American Dietetic Association disclaims responsibility for the application of the information contained herein.

Dedicated to my late husband, Shad,
who encouraged me to write this handbook.

Preface

The purpose of this handbook is to acquaint health care professionals with drug and diet combinations that impose risk of unwanted outcomes. These unwanted outcomes include a reduction of the intended effect of a drug, impairment of nutritional status, and development of a toxic reaction. The handbook is also intended to teach dietitians about clinical problems and abnormal laboratory tests that may result from such drug and nutrient interactions. The handbook is problem-oriented in that the focus is on drug and nutrient interactions and their outcomes in patients having specific types of disease (diabetics, cardiac patients, arthritic patients, etc.). The rationale for this approach is that it has been demonstrated that risk of drug and nutrient interactions is related to the disease characteristics of the patient, which influence the drugs and the diets prescribed, as well as the forms in which food and drugs are administered. The drugs for which interactions and outcomes of interactions are provided are those drugs currently in common use.

Users of the handbook will have the opportunity to select from several cross-indexing systems to check drug groups or individual drugs by generic or brand name, for food and nutrient interactions, and for the beneficial as well as adverse effects of these interactions. They will also be able to check the relative risk of use of particular drug combinations or drug-diet combinations by different patient groups, and they will thereby be able to assess the risk of drug and nutrient interactions in specific patient populations.

Algorithms are employed so that dietitians using the handbook will learn to ask the right questions in examining the risk of drug and nutrient interactions in their own patients.

Changes made from the previous edition include additional information on new drugs, alterations in the Intervention Index (Appendix A), modification of the Algorithms section to facilitate use, and also changes in the section intended to be used by dietitians in counseling patients.

Appendices E, F, and G have been added to this new edition of the handbook, providing information on adverse effects of high-dose vitamin supplements, therapeutic ranges for drugs, and acceptable values for serum levels of nutrients that may be reduced by drug intake.

References are selected to include only reliable sources in which substantive evidence is provided that the interaction is more than a rare event. The references have been revised to update information on drugs previously listed, as well as new drugs.

Our overall intent is to provide a handbook that can readily be used by dietitians who lack knowledge of pharmacology, but who are required to identify and document drug and nutrient interactions in hospital patients.

Also new to this edition is a continuing education (CE) module. The CE module has been approved by the Commission on Dietetic Registration for 3 hours for registered dietitians. This module also serves as an excellent tutorial on how to use the handbook effectively.

Reproducible masters containing patient information on common drugs, including reason for use and guidelines on safe usage to prevent drug-nutrient interactions, are available as a supplement to this handbook. The patient information within the handbook is detailed and is intended for use in counseling. It is suggested that this edition of the handbook be used with the 1992 Drug-Nutrient Interaction Checklist and Screen, in the *Nutrition Interventions Manual* of the Nutrition Screening Initiative.[1]

Acknowledgment

I would like to express my thanks to my secretary, Beverly Hastings, for all her help in preparing the material in this text for publication.

---

[1]*Nutrition Interventions Manual for Professionals Caring for Older Americans.* Washington, DC: Nutrition Screening Initiative; 1992:71-84.

For more information, contact the Nutrition Screening Initiative, 1010 Wisconsin Ave., NW, Suite 800, Washington, DC 20007; 202/625-1662.

How to Use the Handbook

In this handbook, drug and nutrient interactions are grouped according to the type of disease in which they are likely to occur. Within these disease categories, they are listed under the drug(s) used to treat the primary disease and/or its complications. Users of the handbook can check for the risk of a drug and nutrient interaction in a particular type of patient receiving a single drug or a drug combination commonly employed to control the disease present. Users can also check the type of diet, diet change, or dietary supplement that is likely to affect the efficacy or safety of a prescribed drug.

Disease groups for which drug-nutrient interactions are described in the handbook include those of the cardiovascular, respiratory, gastrointestinal, endocrine, neuropsychiatric, musculoskeletal, and genitourinary systems. In addition, drug-nutrient interactions associated with drugs used in the systemic treatment of common dermatoses, infections, and neoplastic disease are included.

Dietitians who wish to inform themselves about desirable and undesirable drug levels can find this information in Appendix F. Those wishing to check blood levels of nutrients in their patients' medical records for changes associated with drug intake can find this information in Appendix E.

The system of cross-referencing, used at the end of the handbook, allows the user to locate symptoms that a particular patient might be experiencing, to determine whether they might be drug-related.

If drug and nutrient interactions have occurred, the appropriate interventions can be found in the Intervention section (Appendix A). You may be further assisted in finding medication-related interventions for older adults by consulting the 1992 *Nutrition Interventions Manual for Professionals Caring for Older Americans* of the Nutrition Screening Initiative, Washington, DC.

This handbook is meant to be kept in your pocket for use when you counsel patients on how they should take their medications safely, and when you are concerned that particular symptoms could be due to such interactions. The following examples will clarify how to use the handbook in differing clinical situations.

Example A: You have an asthmatic patient whom you will soon be counseling on the risk of drug and nutrient interactions associated with the long-acting theophylline preparation that he has been prescribed. Look up "theophylline" in the respiratory disease section of the handbook. Here you will find that there is a risk of loss of effectiveness of the drug if a change is made to a high-protein diet, and also a risk of drug toxicity if the drug is taken with a high-fat meal. When the patient arrives, these potential problems can be discussed and the patient can be given the handout on theophylline.

Example B: A patient of yours who has diabetes and is receiving an oral antidiabetic drug complains of repeated attacks of flushing. She wants to know if the flushing could be related to the medication; she tells you she is taking chlorpropamide. You could look up "flush" in the index of symptoms at the end of the handbook; this would tell you that chlorpropamide causes flushing. Now look up chlorpropamide in the Diabetes section of the handbook and you will find out that the flushing associated with this drug is related to alcohol consumption. The patient can then be counseled to avoid alcohol.

Continuing Education Module

The CE module includes general information on drug-food and drug-nutrient interactions. This is followed by case studies and a quiz designed to familiarize you with the various ways the handbook can be used and the type of information it contains. The module provides 3 hours of approved continuing education credit for registered dietitians.

Client Education Reproducible Masters

Patient information on reducing the risk of drug and nutrient interactions is provided for 26 commonly prescribed drugs in the form of reproducible masters. General information is provided, along with medication-specific recommendations. Every attempt has been made to produce these materials at the lowest reading level possible and in as simple a format as possible. For information about ordering Patient Education Materials: Supplement to the *Handbook on Drug and Nutrient Interactions,* call ADA's customer service department at 800/745-0775.

The team approach to patient education on drug-nutrient interaction is very common and usually quite effective. The team often includes representatives from nursing, pharmacy, and nutrition services. It is hoped that the patient information provided with this handbook will serve as a starting point for your team approach to drug-nutrient patient education.

Contents

Section I
Cardiovascular Disease

SECTION

I

CARDIOVASCULAR DISEASE

I.1.

CONGESTIVE HEART FAILURE

A. *Drugs used in primary disease control*

GENERIC NAME	BRAND NAME	ASSOCIATED DNI	REFERENCE
Digoxin (Cardiac stimulant)	**Lanoxin** (Burroughs Wellcome)	Anorexia and nausea leading to low food intake & weight loss.	1

B. *Drugs used to treat secondary conditions*

(including diuretics to treat edema, antiarrhythmic drugs, and antianginal drugs)

GENERIC NAME	BRAND NAME	ASSOCIATED DNI	REFERENCE
Furosemide (Loop diuretic)	**Lasix** (Hoechst-Roussel)	Hyponatremia.	2
		Hypokalemia and digitalis. toxicity	3
		Hypomagnesia; calcium loss.	4,5
		Thiamin depletion.	6

GENERIC NAME	BRAND NAME	ASSOCIATED DNI	REFERENCE
Bumetanide (Loop diuretic)	**Bumex** (Roche)	See furosemide.	
Ethacrynic acid (Loop diuretic)	**Edecrin** (Merck Sharp Dohme, MSD)	See furosemide.	
Amiloride (K+-sparing diuretic)	**Midamor** (MSD)	Hyponatremia.	7
		Hyperkalemia. Anorexia.	8
Spironolactone (K+-sparing diuretic)	**Aldactone** (Searle)	Hyponatremia.	9
		Hyperkalemia.	
Triamterene (K+-sparing diuretic)	**Dyrenium** (Smith Kline French, SKF)	Hyperkalemia. Folate depletion.	10,11
Quinidine (Anti-arrhythmic)	**Duraquin** (Parke-Davis) **Cardioquin** (Purdue-Frederick)	Vitamin K deficiency if given with anticoagulants.	12
		Quinidine toxicity may be precipitated by high intake of citrus fruit juices. Signs are fast, irregular pulse, vomiting, diarrhea, and loss of consciousness.	
Encainide (Anti-arrhythmic)	**Enkaid** (Bristol Labs)	Hyperglycemia in diabetics. Anorexia & nausea are signs of toxicity.	13,14
Procainamide (Anti-arrhythmic)	**Procan SR** (Parke Davis)	Anorexia, nausea & vomiting may occur.	15

GENERIC NAME	BRAND NAME	ASSOCIATED DNI	REFERENCE
		Risk of toxicity is higher in geriatric patients.	16
Amiodarone (Anti-arrhythmic)	**Cordarone** (Wyeth)	Weight gain due to hypothyroidism is reported in 2–10% of patients. Anorexia and nausea are common.	17
Nitroglycerin (NTG) (Antianginal)	**Nitro Bid** (Marion)	Faintness may occur with NTG and other nitrates, worse when taken with alcohol.	18

Risk factors for adverse effects of cardiac drugs related to drug and nutrient interactions

1. Related to drug regimen: Risk of slowed absorption of digoxin is increased by bran cereal breakfast food. If bran cereal is eaten, the patient should be advised to take the digoxin at an alternate time of the day.
2. Related to diet: Risk of weight loss due to digoxin is increased in patients whose diets are hypocaloric. Risk of arrhythmia due to digoxin toxicity is high in patients whose diets are low in potassium.
3. Related to disease: Risk of weight loss due to digoxin is increased in anorexic patients with severe congestive heart failure and in those with renal impairment.
4. Related to fluids: If the patient is receiving loop diuretics and becomes dehydrated, hypernatremia may occur with congestive heart failure.
5. Related to alcohol consumption: Faintness with nitroglycerin is more common and more severe if alcohol is consumed. Alcohol consumption should be avoided with these cardiac drugs.

I.2.

THROMBOSES

A. *Drugs used in primary disease control*

GENERIC NAME	BRAND NAME	ASSOCIATED DNI	REFERENCE
Warfarin (Anticoagulant)	**Coumadin** (DuPont)	Bleeding due to antivitamin K effect.	1
	Panwarfarin (Abbott)	Vitamin K in formula foods or diets high in vitamin K may reduce anti-coagulant effect. It is important to maintain a consistent level of vitamin K intake in the diet.	2

Risk factors for adverse outcomes of interactions of anticoagulants and nutrients

1. Vitamin E, given as a supplement, may increase the anticoagulant effect of warfarin and cause bleeding.
2. Anticoagulant effects of warfarin and related drugs are increased by intake of herbal teas containing coumarin.
3. Anticoagulant effect of warfarin and related drugs is increased by concurrent use of antibiotics and a diet lacking in green vegetables that contain vitamin K. Antibiotics known to increase the anticoagulant effect of warfarin and related drugs include moxalactam, cefamandole, cefotetan, and cefoperazone.
4. The anticoagulant effect of warfarin and related drugs is reduced by concurrent intake of very large amounts of vitamin K from vegetables and by intake of significant levels of vitamin K in formula foods.

B. *Drugs used for prevention of secondary conditions*

GENERIC NAME	BRAND NAME	ASSOCIATED DNI	REFERENCE
Pentoxifylline (Lowers blood viscosity)	**Trental** (Hoescht-Roussel)	Anorexia, dry mouth, nausea, dyspepsia.	3

I.3.

ATHEROSCLEROSIS AND HYPERCHOLESTEROLEMIA

A. *Drugs used in primary disease control*

GENERIC NAME	BRAND NAME	ASSOCIATED DNI	REFERENCE
Cholestyramine (Lipid-lowering)	**Questran** (B-M)	High, long-term intake causes folate deficiency & depletion of fat-soluble vitamins, including B-carotene due to malabsorption. Also decreased absorption of B_{12} and folate.	1
		Cholestyramine can also cause hyperchloremic metabolic acidosis, presenting as severe fatigue. Risk of acidosis is highest in those with renal impairment. If constipation occurs, increased fiber and fluids are advised.	2

GENERIC NAME	BRAND NAME	ASSOCIATED DNI	REFERENCE
Colestipol (Lipid-lowering)	**Colestid** (Upjohn)	See cholestyramine.	
Probucol (Lipid-lowering)	**Lorelco** (Merrell Dow)	Absorption is better if given after food. Give with meals.	3
		May cause anorexia & anemia.	4
Gemfibrozil (Lipid-lowering)	**Lopid** (Parke-Davis)	Dry mouth, anorexia & gas after food may occur with this drug.	5
Lovastatin (Lipid-lowering)	**Mevacor** (MSD)	Give with evening meal for maximum effect. May cause mild GI symptoms.	6,7
Clofibrate (Lipid-lowering)	**Atromid-S** (Ayerst)	Nausea, vomiting & gas if given after fatty food that promotes drug absorption.	8
		Increases antivitamin K effect of warfarin & combination can cause bleeding.	9
Niacin (Lipid-lowering vitamin)	**Nicobid** (Armour)	Causes flushing.	10
		Large doses can cause hyperglycemia in diabetics.	11,12

GENERIC NAME	BRAND NAME	ASSOCIATED DNI	REFERENCE
		Slow-release niacin preparations may be hepatotoxic, may impose risk of bone marrow suppression, and may impair thyroid function.	

Risk factors for adverse outcomes of drug and nutrient interactions in patients on lipid-lowering drugs

1. Related to drug regimen: For cholestyramine and colestipol, the risk of vitamin depletion is increased by high dose and prolonged usage.
2. Related to diet: For clofibrate, gemfibrozil, and lovastatin, GI symptoms occur when the drug is given after a meal.
3. Related to drug formulation: Long-acting niacin preparations given at high dosages can be toxic to the liver, bone marrow, and thyroid.

I.4.

HYPERTENSION

A. *Drugs used in primary disease control*

GENERIC NAME	BRAND NAME	ASSOCIATED DNI	REFERENCE
Captopril (ACE-I*)	**Capoten** (Squibb)	Dry mouth, loss of taste, nausea, anorexia, gastritis, weight loss, hypoalbuminemia, and hyperkalemia.	1

*ACE-I = acronym for angiotensin I-converting enzyme inhibitor.

GENERIC NAME	BRAND NAME	ASSOCIATED DNI	REFERENCE
Enalapril (ACE-I)	**Vasotec** (MSD)	Similar to captopril except no loss of taste.	2
Hydralazine (Vasodilator)	**Apresoline** (Ciba)	Drug absorption enhanced by food.	3
		Peripheral neuropathy due to vitamin B_6 deficiency; supplementation should correct.	4
		Tartrazine sensitivity. Avoid licorice.	5
Minoxidil (Vasodilator)	**Loniten** (Upjohn)	Weight gain due to edema.	6
Methyldopa (Antiadrenergic)	**Aldomet** (MSD)	Drug absorption reduced by high protein or by an amino acid meal fed with drug.	7
		Iron salts may reduce anti-hypertensive effect.	8
		Nausea, vomiting, reduced food intake may be due to sore tongue and dry mouth. Malabsorption may occur.	9
Clonidine (Antiadrenergic)	**Catapres** (B-I)	Suppresses signs of hypoglycemia in diabetics.	10
		Reduces food intake due to dry mouth.	11
		Inhibits flushing due to niacin.	12

GENERIC NAME	BRAND NAME	ASSOCIATED DNI	REFERENCE
Guanabenz (Antiadrenergic)	**Wytensin** (Wyeth)	Reduces food intake due to dry mouth or bad taste.	13
Guanethidine (Postganglionic adrenergic blocking agent)	**Ismelin** (Ciba)	Weight gain may occur due to edema.	14
Rauwolfia (Antiadrenergic)	**Serpasil** (Ciba) **Reserpine** (Various) **Raudixin** (Princeton) **Harmonyl** (Abbott) **Rauwiloid** (Riker) **Moderil** (Pfizer)	Anorexia. Weight gain may occur due to edema.	14
Prazosin (α-adrenergic blocking agent)	**Minipress** (Pfizer)	Weight gain may occur due to edema.	15
Propranolol (β-adrenergic blocking agent)	**Inderal** (Ayerst)	Drug uptake enhanced by food.	16
		Hypoglycemia may occur in diabetics on oral agents.	17
		Increases serum triglycerides.	18
		Dose decrease needed if hypo-albuminemic to avoid CNS side effects.	19
Metoprolol (β-adrenergic blocking agent)	**Lopressor** (Geigy)	See propranolol.	

GENERIC NAME	BRAND NAME	ASSOCIATED DNI	REFERENCE
Nadolol (β-adrenergic blocking agent)	**Corgard** (Princeton)	See propranolol.	
Atenolol (β-adrenergic blocking agent)	**Tenormin** (Stuart)	See propranolol.	
Timolol (β-adrenergic blocking agent)	**Blocadren** (MSD)	See propranolol.	
Pindolol (β-adrenergic blocking agent)	**Visken** (Sandoz)	Food does not affect drug absorption.	20
		Drug does not increase triglyceride levels.	21
		Increased weight is due to edema.	
Labetalol (β-adrenergic blocking agent)	**Normodyne** (Schering)	Food increases blood levels of the drug.	22
Hydrochlorothiazide (Thiazide diuretic)	**Esidrix** (Ciba) **HydroDIURIL** (MSD) **Oretic** (Abbott)	Increases potassium loss & risk of hypokalemia/hypomagnesemia.	23
		Increased sodium loss confers risk of hyponatremia.	24
		Increases blood glucose.	25
		Increases blood lipids.	26
		May retard osteoporosis.	27
		Increases uric acid and can potentiate gout.	28

NOTE: These effects can be caused by other thiazides.

GENERIC NAME	BRAND NAME	ASSOCIATED DNI	REFERENCE
Nifedipine (Antianginal)	**Procardia** (Pfizer)	Flushing may occur, which is prevented by a low-fat meal. Should not be taken with grapefruit juice because of risk of rapid pulse and dizziness. Weight gain due to edema is common with this calcium channel blocker.	29,30, 31
Verapamil (Antianginal)	**Calan** (Searle)	Calcium supplements may decrease effect of this and other calcium channel blockers. Verapamil inhibits elimination and prolongs effects of alcohol intoxication.	24,25
Diltiazem (Antianginal)	**Cardizem** (Marion)	See information on Verapamil.	
Felodipine (Calcium channel blocker)	**Plendil** (MSD)	See nifedipine for risk of taking with grapefruit juice.	

Risk factors related to adverse outcomes of drug and nutrient interactions for patients on antihypertensive agents

1. Related to drug regimen: For methyldopa, risk of inadequate antihypertensive effect due to poor drug absorption is greatest

when the drug is given with iron, with a high-protein meal, or with a protein hydrolysate.

2. Related to diet: Risk of hyponatremia and hypokalemia with thiazides is greater in patients on sodium-restricted and low-potassium diets. The risk of weight gain due to fluid retention in patients on rauwolfia drugs, guanethidine, and prazosin is greatest in patients who have a high sodium intake. Weight loss associated with loss of taste in patients taking captopril is greatest if the patient is also taking digoxin.
3. Related to disease state: For thiazides, the risk of hyperglycemia is greater in diabetics; risk of hyperlipidemia is greater in diabetics, in those with genetic disorders of lipid metabolism, and in those on isotretinoin for acne. Hypercalcemia, which may occur with prolonged thiazide intake, may suggest a parathyroid tumor. Thiazide-induced hypercalcemia may occur in renal disease and vitamin D intoxication where hypercalcemia is already present; it may then be exacerbated.

   With hydralazine, the risk of vitamin B_6 deficiency causing neuritis is greatest if the drug is given to a patient with tuberculosis who is already taking isoniazid (a vitamin B_6 antagonist), or to a patient with rheumatoid arthritis who is taking penicillamine (vitamin B_6).
4. Related to age: Advanced age, which in itself may decrease taste perception, increases the risk that loss of taste due to captopril will lead to disinterest in food and reduced food intake.

Conditions contributing to risk of important DNI

1. Loss of taste due to captopril is likely with high doses in the elderly.
2. Vitamin B_6 deficiency due to hydralazine is likely with concurrent use of isoniazid or other vitamin B_6 antagonist drugs, including penicillamine, and low dietary vitamin B_6 intake.
3. Weight gain due to prazosin, which is associated with salt and water retention, is likely with a high sodium intake.

SECTION I.1 REFERENCES

1. Morrison WL, Edwards RHT. Cardiac cachexia. *Br Med J.* 1991;302:301–302.
2. Lye MDW. Cardiovascular system-diuretics. In: Brocklehurst JC, ed. *Geriatric Pharmacology and Therapeutics.* London: Blackwell Scientific Publ; 1984:87–92.
3. Steiness E. Diuretics, digitalis and arrhythmias. *Acta Med Scand.* 1981; 647(suppl):75–85.
4. Roe DA. Drug-induced mineral depletion in the elderly. In: Roe DA, ed. *Drugs and Nutrition in the Geriatric Patient.* New York: Churchill Livingstone; 1984:114–115.
5. Eknoyan G, Suki WN, Martinez-Maldonardo N. Effect of diuretics on urinary excretion of phosphate, calcium and magnesium in thyroparathyroidectomized dogs. *J Lab Clin Med.* 1970;76:25–28.
6. Seligmann H, Halkin H, Rauschfleisch S, Kaufmann N, Tal R, Motro M, Vered Z, Ezra D. Thiamine deficiency in patients with congestive heart failure receiving long-term furosemide therapy: a pilot study. *Am J Med.* 1991; 91:151–155.
7. Jamieson NJ. Hyponatraemia. *Br Med J.* 1985;290:1723–1728.
8. *Drug Facts and Comparisons.* St. Louis: JB Lippincott Co; 1992:543–545.
9. *Drug Facts and Comparisons.* 1992:546–548.
10. Dorph S, Olgaard A. Effect of triamterene on serum potassium and serum creatinine in long-term treatment with thiazides. *Nord Med.* 1968;79:516–518.
11. Corcino J, Waxman S, Herbert V. Mechanism of triamterene induced megaloblastosis. *Arch Intern Med.* 1970;73:419–424.
12. *Drug Facts and Comparisons.* 1992:589–593.
13. Salerno DN, Fifield J, Krejci JK, Hodges M. Encainide-induced hyperglycemia. *Am J Med.* 1988;84:39–44.
14. Morganroth J, Hodges M, Ruffy R, Granrud G, Southworth, W. The cooperative encainide trial: efficacy, tolerance and dose findings in chronic severe ventricular ectopy. *Am J Cardiol.* 1982;49:1003.
15. Farmer JA, Young JB. Acute myocardial infarction. In: Rakel, LRE, ed. *Conn's Current Therapy.* Philadelphia: WB Saunders; 1992:269–270.
16. Cusack B, Denham, MJ. Nutritional status and drug disposition in the elderly. In: Roe DA, ed. *Drugs and Nutrition in the Geriatric Patient.* 1984:71–91.
17. Lye MDW. Cardiovascular system—treatment of arrhythmias. In: *Geriatric Pharmacology and Therapeutics.* 1984.
18. *Drug Facts and Comparisons.* 1992:580–584.

SECTION I.2 REFERENCES

1. *United States Pharmacopeia Drug Index (USPDI).* 8th ed. Rockville, Md: US Pharmacopeial Convention, Inc; 1988:259–268.
2. Lee N, Schwartz RN, Sharifi R. Warfarin resistance and vitamin K. *Arch Intern Med.* 1981;94:140–141.
3. *Drug Facts and Comparisons.* 1992:281.

SECTION I.3 REFERENCES

1. Roe DA. *Drug-Induced Nutritional Deficiencies.* 2nd ed. Westport, Conn: AVI Publ Co; 1985:158–159.
2. Scheel PJ, Whelton A, Rossiter K, Watson A. Cholestyramine-induced hyperchloremic metabolic acidosis. *J Clin Pharmacol.* 1992;32:536–538.
3. *USPDI.* 1988:1822–1823.
4. Illingworth DR. Lipid-lowering drugs. *Drugs.* 1987;33:259–279.
5. Houlston R, Quiney J, Watts GF, Lewis B. Gemfibrozil in the treatment of resistant familial hypercholesterolaemia and type III hyperlipoproteinaemia. *J Roy Soc Med.* 1988;81:274–276.
6. *USPDI.* 1988:1104–1105.
7. Lovastatin Study Group III. A multicenter comparison of lovastatin and cholestyramine therapy for severe primary hypercholesterolemia. *JAMA.* 1988; 260:359–366.
8. Houin G, Shastri RA, Barre J, Pinchon B, Tillement JP. Influence of food on the absorption of the p-chlorophenolic ester of chlorophenoxyisobutyric acid in man. *Br J Clin Pharmacol.* 1984;17:341–345.
9. Solomon RB, Rosner F. Massive hemorrhage and death during treatment with clofibrate and warfarin. *New York State J Med.* 1973;73:2002-2004.
10. *Facts and Comparisons.* 1988:18–19.
11. O'Brien T, Silverberg JD, Nguyen TT. Nicotinic acid-induced toxicity associated with cytopenia and decreased levels of thyroxine-binding globulin. *Mayo Clin Proc.* 1992;67:465–468.
12. Alhadeff L, Gualtieri CT, Lipton M. Toxic effects of water soluble vitamins. *Nutr Rev.* 1984;42:33–39.

SECTION I.4 REFERENCES

1. Johnston CI, Arnolda L, Hinatari M. Angiotensin converting enzyme inhibitors in the treatment of hypertension. *Drugs.* 1984;27:271–277.
2. Breckenridge A. Angiotensin converting enzyme inhibitors. *Br Med J.* 1988; 296:618–620.
3. Ludden TM, McNay AM Jr, Lin MS. Clinical pharmacokinetics of hydralazine. *Clin Phamacokinet.* 1982;7:185–205.
4. Raskin NH, Fishman RA. Pyridoxine deficiency due to hydralazine. *N Engl J Med.* 1966;273:1182–1185.
5. *Drug Facts and Comparisons.* 1992:761-764.
6. Lye MDW. Cardiovascular system-treatment of hypertension. In: *Geriatric Pharmacology and Therapeutics.* London: Blackwell Scientific Publ; 1984: 118.
7. Myhre E, Rugstad HE, Hansen T. Clinical pharmacokinetics of methyldopa. *Clin Pharmacokinet.* 1982;7:221–233.
8. Campbell N, Paddock V, Sundaram R. Alteration of methyldopa absorption, metabolism and blood pressure control caused by ferrous sulfate and ferrous gluconate. *Clin Pharmacol Ther.* 1988;43:381–386.

9. Shneerson JN, Gazzard BG. Reversible malabsorption caused by methyldopa. *Br Med J.* 1977;2:1456–1457.
10. Hansten PD. *Drug Interactions.* 5th ed. Philadelphia: Lea and Febiger; 1985: 153.
11. Nickerson M, Ruedy J. Antihypertensive agents and the drug therapy of hypertension. In: Goodman LS, Gilman A, eds, *The Pharmacological Basis of Therapeutics.* 5th ed. New York: Macmillan; 1975:711.
12. Sigroth K. Effect of clonidine on nicotinic acid flushing. *Lancet.* 1974;2:58.
13. *Drug Facts and Comparisons.* 1992:742.
14. *Drug Facts and Comparisons.* 1992:744-748.
15. *Drug Facts and Comparisons.* 1992:759.
16. Melander A, Danielson K, Schersten B, Wahlin E. Enhancement of the bioavailability of propanolol and metoprolol by food. *Clin Pharmacol Therap.* 1977;22:108–112.
17. MacLennan WJ, Shepherd AN, Stevenson IH. *The Elderly.* New York: Springer-Verlag; 1984:47.
18. Weinberger MH. Antihypertensive therapy and lipids: evidence, mechanisms and implications. *Arch Intern Med.* 1985;145:1102–1105.
19. Lye MDW. Cardiovascular system: treatment of hypertension. In: *Geriatric Pharmacology and Therapeutics.* 1984:110–111.
20. Melander A, McLean A. Influence of food intake on presystemic clearance of drugs. *Clin Pharmacokinet.* 1983;8:286–296.
21. Harvengt C, Heller FR, Martiat P, Van Nieuwenhuyze Y. Short-term effects of beta blockers atenolol, nadolol, pindolol and propranolol on lipoprotein metabolism in normolipemic subjects. *J Clin Pharmacol.* 1987;27:475–480.
22. Mantyla R, Allonen H, Kanto J, et al. Effect of food on the bioavailability of labetalol. *Br J Clin Pharmacol.* 1980;9:435.
23. Maronde RF, Milgrom M, Dickey JM. Potassium loss with thiazide therapy. *Am Heart J.* 1969;78:16–21.
24. Ashraf N, Locksley R, Arleff AI. Thiazide-induced hyponatremia associated with death or neurologic damage in outpatients. *Am J Med.* 1981;70:1163–1167.
25. Andersson O. The use of diuretics in modern antihypertensive therapy. *Acta Pharmacol Toxicol.* 1984;54(suppl. 1):79–82.
26. Ames RP, Peacock PB. Serum cholesterol during treatment of hypertension with diuretic drugs. *Arch Intern Med.* 1984;144:710–714.
27. Riis B, Christensen C. Actions of thiazide on vitamin D metabolism: a controlled therapeutic trial in normal women early in the post-menopause. *Metabolism.* 1985;34:421–424.
28. McDonald CJ, Hui SL, Tierney WN. Diuretic-induced laboratory abnormalities that predict ventricular ectopy. *J Chron Dis.* 1986;39:127–135.
29. Bailey DG, Spence JD, Munoz C, Arnold JMO. Interaction of citrus juices with felodipine and nifedipine. *Lancet.* 1991;337:268–269.
30. Reitberg DP, Love SJ, Quercia GT, Zinny MA. Effect of food on nifedipine pharmacokinetics. *Clin Pharmacol Ther.* 1987;42:72–75.
31. Bauer LA, Schumock G, Horn J, Ophelm K. Verapamil inhibits ethanol elimination and prolongs the perception of intoxication. *Clin Pharmacol Therap.* 1992;52:6.

Section
II
Respiratory Disease

SECTION

II RESPIRATORY DISEASE

II.1.

BRONCHIAL ASTHMA (drugs used in bronchial asthma are also used to treat wheezing that occurs in chronic obstructive lung disease)

A. *Drugs used in primary disease control*

GENERIC NAME	BRAND NAME	ASSOCIATED DNI	REFERENCE
Theophylline (Broncho-dilator)	**Slo-Phyllin** (Rorer) **Theolair** (Riker) **Theophyl-225** (McNeil) **Elixophyllin** (Forest) **Theo-24** (Searle) **Somophyllin-T** (Fisons) **Somophyllin-CRT** (Fisons) **Theo-Dur Sprinkle** (Key) **Slo-bid Gyrocaps** (Rorer)	Duration of asthma control reduced by high-protein diet.	1

GENERIC NAME	BRAND NAME	ASSOCIATED DNI	REFERENCE
		High-carbohydrate, low-protein diet slows drug metabolism with risk of side effects (including dizziness, flushing and headache) if drug frequency is not reduced.	2
		High fat intake with the drug increases risk of dizziness due to rapid absorption with slow-release products.	3
		Effects of food on theophylline metabolism vary with the drug formulation.	4
		Rate of drug absorption is slowed following feeds in premature infants.	5
		Concurrent intake of coffee or strong tea increases risk of insomnia and cardiac arrhythmias.	6
		Caffeine taken in any form slows the rate of elimination of theophylline.	7

GENERIC NAME	BRAND NAME	ASSOCIATED DNI	REFERENCE
		Duration of drug effect is less when charcoal-broiled meat is eaten.	8
		Intake of formula foods containing fiber slows drug absorption, but increases total amount of drug absorbed.	9
		Anorexia is a common side effect of theophylline.	10

NOTE: Of the brand names listed, the following are immediate-release products: Slo-Phyllin, Theolair, Theophyl-225, Elixophyllin, and Somophyllin-T. The other listed brands are slow-release products. Certain of the drug-nutrient interaction risks are related to use of the slow-release products (ref 3).

GENERIC NAME	BRAND NAME	ASSOCIATED DNI	REFERENCE
Albuterol (Bronchodilator)	**Alupent** (Boehringer-Ingelheim	May cause hyperglycemia in diabetics.	11
	Proventil (Schering)	Drug-induced hyperglycemia may necessitate reduction in the dose of insulin or oral agent they are taking.	12
Terbutaline (Bronchodilator)	**Brethaire** (Geigy)	May increase need for insulin or increase need for oral agent in diabetics (see albuterol).	

GENERIC NAME	BRAND NAME	ASSOCIATED DNI	REFERENCE
Isoetharine (Bronchodilator)	**Isoetharine HCI** (Roxane) **Dey-Lute** (Dey)	Contains sulfite, which causes acute allergic reactions in persons sensitive to sulfite in foods.	13
Prednisone (Anti-inflammatory glucocorticoid)	**Deltasone** (Upjohn) **Liquid Pred** (Muro) **Orasone** (Reid-Powell)	Weight gain due to drug-induced appetite increase or edema.	14
		Stunting of growth in children.	15
		Hyperglycemia may occur in both nondiabetics and diabetics.	16
		Impaired wound healing is common. An increased calcium intake is recommended in adults to reduce the risk of drug-induced osteoporosis.	16a

NOTE: Other glucocorticoids used orally or as inhalants by asthmatics impose risk of similar side effects.

B. ***Drugs used in the treatment of secondary problems*** *(including cough and allergic rhinitis)*

GENERIC NAME	BRAND NAME	ASSOCIATED DNI	REFERENCE
Cromolyn sodium (Antiallergic)	**Intal** (Fisons)	Nausea.	17
Iodinated glycerol (Expectorant)	**Organidin** (Wallace)	Flush reactions with oral anti-diabetic agents due to the high alcohol content of the product.	18
Potassium iodide (Expectorant)	**Iodo-niacin** (Forest)	Hyperkalemia with potassium supplements or salt substitutes. Flush may occur due to the presence of niacin.	18

Risk factors related to adverse outcomes of drug-food interactions for patients on bronchodilator drugs

1. Related to drug regimen: Whether or not theophylline control of wheezing in asthmatics is adversely affected by food intake depends on the drug preparation used (see ref. 4, Section II.1).
2. Related to diet: High intake of coffee or strong tea with theophylline increases risk of insomnia and cardiac arrhythmias. High fat intake with the drug increases risk of dizziness due to rapid absorption. Risk of decreased duration of action of theophylline is associated with sudden increases in protein intake, intake of high protein-nutrient supplements, and increased intake of charcoal-broiled meats.
3. Related to disease states: For theophylline, the risk of anorexia causing a significant anorectic effect such that food intake is markedly reduced is greatest in patients with severe chronic obstructive lung disease.

Conditions contributing to risk of important drug-nutrient interactions

1. Intake of theophylline by patients with chronic lung disease who are initially malnourished and require nutritional intervention by provision of high-protein foods.
2. Risk of acute sulfite reactions relative to isoetharine is greater in persons reacting to sulfite in foods and in those who have asthma or atopic dermatitis.

II.2.

BRONCHITIS AND PNEUMONIA

A. *Drugs used in primary disease control*

GENERIC NAME	BRAND NAME	ASSOCIATED DNI	REFERENCE
Amoxicillin (Antibiotic)	**Amoxil** (Beecham)	Absorption is promoted by high concurrent fluid intake.	1
Azithromycin (Antibiotic)	**Zithromax** (Pfizer)	Nausea and diarrhea may occur.	2
Erythromycin (Antibiotic)	**Erythrocin** (Abbott) **Ilotycin** (Dista)	Absorption of erythromycin stearate is reduced by food. Nausea & diarrhea may occur.	3
Moxalactam (Antibiotic)	**Moxam** (Lilly)	This cephalosporin antibiotic, as well as cefamandole, cefotetan, and cefoperazone, can cause bleeding due to vitamin K deficiency.	4

GENERIC NAME	BRAND NAME	ASSOCIATED DNI	REFERENCE
Trimethoprim (Antibacterial)	**Bactrim** (Roche)* **Septra** (Burroughs Wellcome)*	Trimethoprim can cause folate depletion. Sulfa in the product can cause anemia.	5
Tetracycline (Antibiotic)	**Achromycin V** (Lederle) **Panmycin** (Upjohn) **Robitet** (Robins) **Sumycin** (Squibb)	Interacts with milk and other dairy products, antacids, calcium and iron supplements, and magnesium-containing laxatives to form nonabsorbable complexes resulting in decreased absorption. Avoid using these one hour before and after dose. May be taken with food if GI irritation.	6
Oxytetracycline (Antibiotic)	**Terramycin** (Pfizer; Roerig)	See tetracycline.	6

*NOTE: These products contain trimethoprim + sulfamethoxazole.

B. *Risk factors related to adverse outcomes of drug and nutrient interactions in patients on antibacterials for bronchitis and pneumonia.*

1. Related to drug regimen: The prescription of specific cephalosporin antibiotics, including moxalactam, cefamandole, and cefoperazone but not other cephalosporin antibiotics, increases risk of hemorrhage due to vitamin K deficiency.

C. *Conditions contributing to risk of important DNI*

1. Intake of cephalosporins such as moxalactam by patients on coumarin anticoagulants.
2. Intake of these cephalosporins, which can induce vitamin K deficiency, by patients with liver disease.
3. The likelihood that trimethoprim will cause folate deficiency is increased in patients who previously subsisted on a low-folate diet and in those taking drugs that are folate antagonists (eg, methotrexate, phenobarbital, phenytoin, or sulfasalazine) or with double-strength (DS) products.

II.3.
PULMONARY TUBERCULOSIS

A. *Drugs used in primary disease control*

GENERIC NAME	BRAND NAME	ASSOCIATED DNI	REFERENCE
Isoniazid (INH) (Antitubercu-losis)	**Nydrazid** (Squibb)	Absorption is inadequate if taken after food.	1
		Absorption lowest if taken with high-carbo-hydrate meals. Give while fasting.	2
		Isoniazid is a vitamin B_6 antagonist, best given with 25 mg B_6/day.	3
		Vitamin B_6 should be used to prevent convulsions in isoniazid overdose cases.	4

GENERIC NAME	BRAND NAME	ASSOCIATED DNI	REFERENCE
		Pellagra can rarely occur secondary to vitamin B_6 deficiency if B_6 is not given.	5
		Interferes with vitamin D metabolism; vitamin D supplement may be required in long-term care patients on isoniazid.	6
Rifampin (Anti-tuberculosis)	**Rifadin** (Merrell Dow)	Risk of osteomalacia.	7
	Rimactane (Ciba)	Inhibits standard tests for folate and vitamin B_{12}.	8
		Food decreases drug absorption; should be given fasting.	9
Pyrazinamide (Antituber-culosis)	**Pyrazinamide** (Lederle)	Neuritis and anemia may occur due to vitamin B_6 deficiency.	10
		Pellagra has also been reported due to pyrazinamide.	11
		These drug-induced vitamin deficiencies can be prevented by giving a vitamin B_6 supplement.	12
Ethambutol (Antituber-culosis)	**Myambutol** (Lederle)	Should be taken with food to avoid nausea.	13

GENERIC NAME	BRAND NAME	ASSOCIATED DNI	REFERENCE
		May precipitate gout.	14
		May induce loss of visual acuity and risk is highest in diabetics not in glycemic control.	15

Risk factors related to adverse outcomes of drug-nutrient interactions for tuberculosis patients

1. Related to drug regimen: Risk of vitamin B_6 deficiency in patients on isoniazid is increased by concurrent intake of other antituberculosis drugs; eg, pyrazinamide also carries this risk. Intake of isoniazid without concurrent intake of a pyridoxine supplement also increases risk. Risk is further increased if the patient is a slow acetylator of isoniazid.
2. Related to diet: Risk of pyridoxine deficiency in patients on isoniazid is greater in patients on very low intakes of vitamin B_6. The risk of pellagra in patients on this drug is present if a very low protein and low niacin diet is consumed.
3. Related to disease state: In patients with advanced tuberculosis requiring prolonged antituberculosis therapy, the risk of drug-induced vitamin B_6 deficiency due to isoniazid is increased.

Conditions contributing to risk of important DNI

1. Vitamin B_6 deficiency due to antituberculosis drugs is more likely in malnourished patients not on B_6 supplements.
2. Risk of osteomalacia due to isoniazid is greater in nonmilk drinkers who are homebound or in institutions.
3. Risk of vitamin D depletion in patients taking isoniazid may be increased by concurrent intake of another antituberculosis drug, rifampin.
4. Risk of vitamin B_6 deficiency due to pyrazinamide is associated with the same deficiency induced by isoniazid, given that the two drugs are taken at the same time.

SECTION II.1 REFERENCES

1. Feldman CH, Hutchinson VE, Pippenger CE, Blumenfeld TA, Feldman BR, Davis WJ. Effect of dietary protein and carbohydrate on theophylline metabolism in children. *Pediatrics.* 1980;66:956–962.
2. Fagan TC, Walle T, Oexmann MJ, Walle UK, Bai SA, Gaffney TE. Increased clearance of propranolol and theophylline by high-protein compared with high carbohydrate diet. *Clin Pharmacol Ther.* 1987;41:402–406.
3. Vaughan L, Milavetz G, Hill M, Weinberger M, Hendeles L. Food-induced dose-dumping of Theo-24, a "once daily" theophylline product. *Drug Intell Clin Pharm.* 1984;18:510.
4. Hendeles L, Iafrate RP, Weinberger M. A clinical and pharmacokinetic basis for the selection and use of slow-release theophylline products. *Clin Pharmacokinet.* 1984;9:95–135.
5. Heimann G, Murgescu J, Bergt U. Influence of food intake on bioavailability of theophylline in premature infants. *Eur J Clin Pharmacol.* 1982;22:171–173.
6. Jonkman JHG, Upton RA. Pharmacokinetic drug interactions with theophylline. *Clin Pharmacokinet.* 1984;9:309–324.
7. Jonkman JHG, Sollie FAE, Sauter T, Steinijans VW. The influence of caffeine on the steady-state pharmacokinetics of theophylline. *Clin Pharmacol Ther.* 1991;49:248–255.
8. Alvares AP. Environmental influences on drug biotransformation in humans. *World Rev Nutr Dietet.*1984;43:45–59.
9. Roe DA. A comparison of drug-nutrient and nutrient-nutrient interactions. In: Bodwell CE, Erdman JW, eds, *Nutrient Interactions.* NY: Marcel Dekker, Inc; 1988:365–377.
10. *USPDI.* 1988:533–543.
11. MacLennan WJ, Shepherd AN, Stevenson IH. *The Elderly.* Berlin, NY: Springer-Verlag; 1984:64–65.
12. Smith AP, Banks J, Cheong, B, Gunawardena. Mechanisms of abnormal glucose metabolism during the treatment of acute severe asthma. *Quart J Med.* 1992;NS82:71–80.
13. *Facts and Comparisons.* 1988:696.
14. Roe DA. Drug and nutrient interactions. In: Schneider HA, Anderson CE, Coursin DB, eds, *Nutritional Support of Medical Practice.* 2nd ed. Philadelphia: Harper & Row; 1983:320–327.
15. Niermann WA, Van Meter TE Jr. Efficacy of Medrol in treating bronchial asthma in children. *Metabolism.* 1958;7:473–476.
16. Davis PJ, Davis FB. Control of blood sugar level in elderly diabetic patients. *Primary Care.* 1982;9:45–51.

16a. Roe DA. *Drug and Diet Interactions.* New York: Van Nostrand Reinhold; 1989:91.

17. *Facts and Comparisons.* 1988:729–730.
18. *Facts and Comparisons.* 1988:760–762.

SECTION 11.2 REFERENCES

1. Welling PG, Huang H, Koch PA. et al. Bioavailability of ampicillin and amoxicillin in fasted and non-fasting subjects. *J Pharm Sci.* 1977;66:549–552.
2. *Drug Facts and Comparisons.* 1992:2693.
3. Viswanathan CT, Welling PG. Food effects on drug absorption in the elderly. In: Roe DA, ed. *Drugs and Nutrition in the Geriatric Patient.* New York: Churchill Livingstone; 1984:47–70.
4. Shearer MJ, Bechtold H, Andrassy K, Koderisch J, McCarthy, PT, Trenk D, Jahnchen E, Ritz E. Mechanism of cephalosporin-induced hypoprothrombinemia: relation to cephalosporin side chain, vitamin K metabolism, and vitamin K status. *J Clin Pharmacol.* 1988;28:88–95.
5. Girdwood RH, DaCosta AJ, Samson RR. Co-trimoxazole as a possible cause of folate depletion. *Br J Haematol.* 1973;25:279–280.
6. Clayman CB, ed. *AMA Guide to Prescription and Over-the-Counter Drugs.* New York: Random House; 1988.

SECTION II.3 REFERENCES

1. Melander A, Danielson K, Hanson A, Jansson L, Rerup C, Schersten B, Thulin T, Wahlin E. Reduction of isoniazid bioavailability in normal men by concomitant intake of food. *Acta Med Scand.* 1976;200:93–97.
2. Holdiness MR. Clinical pharmacokinetics of the antituberculosis drugs. *Clin Pharmacokinet.* 1984;9:511–544.
3. Jones WA, Penrhyn Jones G. Peripheral neuropathy due to isoniazid. *Lancet.* 1953;1:1073–1074.
4. Katz GA, Jobin GC. Large doses of pyridoxine in the treatment of massive ingestion of isoniazid. *Am Rev Resp Dis.* 1970;101:991–992.
5. Bender DA, Russell-Jones R. Isoniazid-induced pellagra. *Lancet.* 1979;2: 1125–1126.
6. Brodie MJ, Boobis AR, Hillyard CJ, Abeyasekera G, Stevenson JC, MacIntyre I, Kevin Park B. Effect of rifampicin and isoniazid on vitamin D metabolism. *Clin Pharmacol Therap.* 1982;32:525–530.
7. Brodie MJ, Hillyard CJ. Calcium metabolism during rifampicin and isoniazid therapy for tuberculosis. *J Roy Soc Med.* 1982;75:919.
8. *Facts and Comparisons.* 1988:1540.
9. Acocella G. Clinical pharmacokinetics of rifampicin. *Clin Pharmacokinet.* 1978;3:108–127.
10. McCurdy PR, Donohoe RF, McGovern M. Reversible sideroblastic anemia caused by pyrazinoic acid (pyrazinamide). *Ann Intern Med.* 1966;64:1280-1284.
11. Jorgensen J. Pellagra probably due to pyrazinamide: development during combined therapy for tuberculosis. *Int J Dermatol.* 1983;22:44–45.
12. Roe DA. *Drug-Induced Nutritional Deficiencies.* 2nd ed. Westport, Conn: AVI Publ Co; 1985:287–288.
13. *Facts and Comparisons.* 1988.
14. *USPDI.* 1988:1048.
15. MacLennan WJ, Shepherd AN, Stevenson IH. *The Elderly.* 1984:68.

Section

III

Gastrointestinal Disease

SECTION

III GASTROINTESTINAL DISEASE

III.1. PEPTIC ULCER

A. *Drugs used in primary disease control*

GENERIC NAME	BRAND NAME	ASSOCIATED DNI	REFERENCE
Cimetidine (H^2 receptor antagonist)	**Tagamet** (SKF)	Can induce vitamin B_{12} depletion.	1
		Increases risk of bleeding associated with warfarin-induced vitamin K deficiency.	2
		May increase risk of intoxication due to increase in blood alcohol levels.	3
		Antacids given with this or with other H receptor antagonists, to treat gastritis, inhibit drug absorption.	4

GENERIC NAME	BRAND NAME	ASSOCIATED DNI	REFERENCE
		Spacing of H[2] receptor antagonist and antacid has been recommended, to avoid this effect; but if cimetidine is given, an antacid is not usually required.	
Ranitidine (H[2] receptor antagonist)	**Zantac** (Glaxo)	Risk of vitamin B_{12} depletion and of potentiation of warfarin-induced bleeding as for cimetidine.	5
Famotidine (H[2] receptor antagonist)	**Pepcid** (MSD)	Risk of vitamin B12 depletion expected as for cimetidine, but not cited in standard references.	6
		No risk of bleeding due to warfarin.	7
Omeprazole (Antisecretory drug)	**Prilosec** (MSD)	May cause dry mouth and anorexia.	8
Misoprostol (Antisecretory drug)	**Cytotec** (Searle)	May cause nausea, dyspepsia, and diarrhea.	9
Sodium bicarbonate (Antacid)	**Alka-Seltzer** (Miles)	Each tablet (2/dose) contains 284 mg sodium. High intake imposes risk of congestive heart failure in cardiac patients.	10

GENERIC NAME	BRAND NAME	ASSOCIATED DNI	REFERENCE
		May cause milk alkali syndrome if taken in large amounts with milk: signs are hypercalcemia and renal failure.	11
		High intake reduces absorption of folic acid.	12
Aluminum hydroxide (Antacid)	**Amphojel** (Wyeth-Ayerst) **Maalox** (Rorer) **Di-Gel** (Plough)	Interferes with drug absorption by causing increase in GI and in urinary pH and by drug binding. Decreased absorption of tetracycline.	13
		Hypophosphatemia and secondary osteomalacia may occur with abuse of these and other aluminum hydroxide-containing antacids.	14
Calcium carbonate (Antacid)	**TUMS** (Norcliff-Thayer)	May reduce iron absorption.	15
		High intake imposes risk of milk-alkali syndrome.	11

GENERIC NAME	BRAND NAME	ASSOCIATED DNI	REFERENCE
Magnesium hydroxide (Antacid)	**M.O.M.** (Ulmer)	Magnesium toxicity can develop in renal failure patients.	16
Sucralfate (Anti-ulcer)	**Carafate** (Marion)	May reduce drug absorption. Side effects include constipation, GI discomfort, and hypophosphatemia.	17

B. ***Drugs used to treat secondary conditions***
(includes drugs used to treat gastroesophageal reflux and to assist in ulcer healing)

GENERIC NAME	BRAND NAME	ASSOCIATED DNI	REFERENCE
Metoclopramide (antireflux)	**Reglan** (Robins)	In diabetics, rate of drug and nutrient absorption from the intestine may be increased, including glucose. Nausea, decreased intake.	18
Propantheline bromide (Anti-secretory)	**Pro-Banthine** (Searle)	Promotes absorption of riboflavin and of drugs that are better absorbed when gastric emptying is slowed.	19
		Causes dry mouth.	10

Risk factors related to adverse outcomes of drug-nutrient interactions for peptic ulcer patients

1. Risk of vitamin B_{12} depletion in patients on cimetidine or ranitidine is increased if either drug is taken by vegans for an extended time (>1 yr).
2. A risk has been defined for the development of a milk-alkali syndrome in patients taking high doses of calcium carbonate and having advanced renal disease.
3. Sucralfate can lead to significant hypophosphatemia.

III.2.
CYSTIC FIBROSIS

A. *Drugs used in primary disease control*

GENERIC NAME	BRAND NAME	ASSOCIATED DNI	REFERENCE
Pancrelipase (Digestive enzymes)	**Pancrease** (McNeil) **Cotazym-S** (Organon)	Decreases the steatorrhea due to cystic fibrosis.	1
	Viokase (Robins)	May decrease the absorption of folate if given with H^2 receptor antagonist, which is used to lessen inactivation of the digestive enzymes.	2
Gentamicin (Antibiotic)	**Garamycin** (Schering)	Nephrotoxic; may induce potassium and magnesium depletion.	3

B. ***Drugs used for the treatment of secondary problems*** (includes sodium depletion and vitamin deficiencies)

GENERIC NAME	BRAND NAME	ASSOCIATED DNI	REFERENCE
Sodium chloride (Electrolyte replacement)	**Slo-salt** (Nission)	Used to offset excess sodium and chloride losses in sweat.	4
Vitamin A (Fat-soluble vitamin)	**Aquasol A** (Armour)	May cause signs of vitamin A toxicity if dose exceeds 10,000 IU/day.	5

III.3.
INFLAMMATORY BOWEL DISEASE

A. *Drugs used in primary disease control*

GENERIC NAME	BRAND NAME	ASSOCIATED DNI	REFERENCE
Sulfasalazine (GI-anti-inflammatory)	**Azulfidine** (Pharmacia)	May induce folate deficiency; risk is highest in patients with malabsorption.	1
Olsalazine (GI-anti inflammatory)	**Dipentum** (Pharmacia)	May cause diarrhea.	2
Prednisone (Corticosteroid)	**Deltasone** (Upjohn)	Risk of osteoporosis with high or prolonged usage. See also side effects described for asthma.	3

B. ***Drugs used to treat secondary conditions***
(includes drugs used to treat diarrhea)

GENERIC NAME	BRAND NAME	ASSOCIATED DNI	REFERENCE
Diphenoxylate w/ atropine (Antidiarrheal)	**Lomotil** (Searle)	May cause dry mouth.	4
Loperamide (Antidiarrheal)	**Imodium** (Janssen)	Controls diarrhea but risk is of electrolyte imbalance.	5

Risk factors related to adverse outcomes of drug-nutrient interactions for patients on drugs to control inflammatory bowel disease

1. Risk factors for folate deficiency in patients on sulfasalazine include low intake of dietary folate sources (vegetables, fortified cereals), malabsorption and concurrent intake of other drugs that adversely affect folate utilization (phenytoin).
2. Risk factors for osteoporosis in patients with inflammatory bowel disease include high daily intake of prednisone or other corticosteroids by a patient with a low calcium intake (<500 mg/day).

III.4.
CONSTIPATION

A. ***Drugs used in primary disease control***

GENERIC NAME	BRAND NAME	ASSOCIATED DNI	REFERENCE
Magnesium sulfate (Saline cathartic)	**Epsom salts**	Can cause severe dehydration and hypermag-nesemia.	1

GENERIC NAME	BRAND NAME	ASSOCIATED DNI	REFERENCE
Phenolphthalein (Laxative)	**Correctol** (Plough) **Ex-Lax** (Sandoz) **Feen-a-Mint** (Plough)	Abuse of this drug can cause potassium depletion and malabsorption with weight loss.	2
Bisacodyl (Laxative)	**Dulcolax** (Boehringer)	See phenolphthalein.	
Senna (Laxative)	**Senokot** (Purdue-Frederick)	See phenolphthalein.	

B. ***Drugs used to treat secondary conditions***
(Includes stool softeners and emollient laxatives)

GENERIC NAME	BRAND NAME	ASSOCIATED DNI	REFERENCE
Mineral oil (Emollient laxative)	**Kondremul** (Fisons) **Agoral** (Parke-Davis)	Reduces absorption of fat-soluble vitamin deficiency with long-term use.	3
Psyllium gum (Bulking agent)	**Metamucil** (Procter and Gamble)	Can reduce appetite. Reduces absorption of riboflavin.	4 5

Risk Factors

Risk factors for malabsorption due to laxatives include laxative abuse and, in the case of mineral oil, intake of the mineral oil at or close to the time when sources of fat-soluble vitamins are ingested.

1. Due to the drug regimen: Risk factors for mineral and particularly potassium depletion due to laxatives are related to laxative abuse.
2. Due to the diet regimen: Risk factors for mineral depletion and for malnutrition secondary to malabsorption of vitamins include, in addition to taking mineral oil at the same time as food is ingested, intake of a diet that is marginal or deficient in the vitamins of interest.

3. Due to the disease: Risk factors for mineral depletion due to laxatives include the anorexia-bulimia syndrome and paranoid state in which laxative abuse is most common.

SECTION III.1 REFERENCES

1. Streeter AN, Goulston KJ, Bathur FA, Hilmer RS, Crane GG, Pheils MT. Cimetidine and malabsorption of cobalamin. *Dig Dis Sci.* 1982;27:13–16.
2. Somogyi A, Gugler R. Drug interactions with cimetidine. *Clin Pharmacokinet.* 1982;7:23–41.
3. Feely J, Wood AJJ. Effects of cimetidine on the elimination and actions of alcohol. *JAMA.* 1982;247:2819–2821.
4. Steinberg WN, Lewis JH, Katz DM. Antacids inhibit absorption of cimetidine. *N Engl J Med.* 1982;307:400–403.
5. Kirch W, Hoensch H, Janosch HD. Interactions and non-interactions with ranitidine. *Clin Pharmacokinet.* 1984;9:493–510.
6. *USPDI.* 1988:1089–1091.
7. *Facts and Comparisons.* 1988:1277.
8. *Drug Facts and Comparisons.* 1992:1535–1540.
9. *Drug Facts and Comparisons.* 1992:1532–1534.
10. *Facts and Comparisons.* 1988:1280–1281.
11. Levy G, Gibaldi M, Procknal JA. Effect of an anticholinergic agent on the absorption of riboflavin. *J Pharm Sci.* 1972; 61:798–799.
12. *Facts and Comparisons.* 1988:1256-1261.
13. Roe DA. Adverse nutritional effects of OTC drug use in the elderly. In: *Drugs and Nutrition in the Geriatric Patient.* 1984:122–133.
14. Randall RE Jr, Strauss MB, McNeeley WF. The milk-alkali syndrome. *Arch Intern Med.* 1961;107:163-181.
15. MacKenzie JF, Russell RJ. The effect of pH on folic acid absorption. *Clin Sci Molec Med.* 1976; 51:363-368.
16. Hansten PD. *Drug Interactions.* 5th ed. Philadelphia: Lea and Febiger; 1985: 238, 356–357.
17. Insogna KL, Bordley DR, Caro JF, Lockwood DH. Osteomalacia and weakness from excessive antacid. *JAMA.* 1980:2544–2546.
18. Coste JF, et al. In vitro interactions of oral hematinics and antacid suspensions. *Curr Ther Res.* 1977;22:205–206.
19. Wacker WEC, Parisi AF. Magnesium metabolism. *N Engl J. Med.* 1968;278: 712–717, 771–776.
20. *Facts and Comparisons.* 1988:1251.

SECTION III.2 REFERENCES

1. Rylance G, ed. *Drugs for Children.* Copenhagen: WHO Regional Office for Europe; 1987:78–79.

2. Russell RN, Ohar GJ, Dutta SK, Rosenberg IH. Influence of intraluminal pH on folate absorption: studies in control subjects and in patients with pancreatic insufficiency. *J Lab Clin Med.* 1979;93:428–436.
3. Bar RS, Wilson HE, Mazzaferri EL. Hypomagnesemic hypocalcemia secondary to renal magnesium wasting: a possible consequence of high dose gentamicin therapy. *Ann Intern Med.* 1975;82:646-648.
4. Roe DA. Drug interference with the assessment of nutritional status. *Clin Lab Med.* 1981;1:647–664.
5. Roe DA. *Diet and Drug Interactions.* New York: Van Nostrand Reinhold; 1988:113–115.

SECTION III.3 REFERENCES

1. Swinson CM, Perry J, Lumb M, Levi AJ. Role of sulfasalazine in the aetiology of folate deficiency in ulcerative colitis. *Gut.* 1981;22:456–461.
2. Shanahan F, Targan S. Medical treatment of inflammatory bowel disease. *Ann Rev Med.* 1992;43:125–133.
3. Roe DA. *Diet and Drug Interactions.* 1988:91.
4. Brocklehurst JC. Gastrointestinal system. In: Brocklehurst JC, ed. *Geriatric Pharmacology and Therapeutics.* Oxford, London: Blackwell Sci Publ; 1984: 215–216.
5. *Facts and Comparisons.* 1988:1323.

SECTION III.4 REFERENCES

1. Ditzler JW. Epsom salts poisoning and a review of magnesium ion physiology. *Anesthesiology.* 1970;32:378–380.
2. Fleming BJ, Genuth SM, Gould AB, Kamionkowski MD. Laxative-induced hypokalemia, sodium depletion and hyperreninemia. *Ann Intern Med.* 1975;83:60–62.
3. Curtis AC, Ballmer RS. The prevention of carotene absorption by liquid petrolatum. *JAMA.* 1939;113:1785–1788.
4. Roe DA, Kalkwarf H, Stevens J. Effect of fiber supplements on the apparent absorption of pharmacological doses of riboflavin. *J Am Diet Assoc.*1988;88: 211–213.

Section IV Endocrine Disease

SECTION
IV
ENDOCRINE DISEASE

IV.I.
DIABETES MELLITUS

A. *Drugs used in primary disease control*

GENERIC NAME	BRAND NAME	ASSOCIATED DNI	REFERENCE
Insulin (Anti-diabetic agent)	**Humulin R** (Lilly)	Can cause hypoglycemia.	1
		Can increase appetite.	2
Chlorpropamide (Antidiabetic)	**Diabinese** (Pfizer)	Can cause hypoglycemia.	3
		Flush reaction may occur when taken with alcohol.	4
		Weight gain may occur due to fluid retention or increased appetite and food intake.	5
		Risk of CHD may be increased.	6
		Higher risk of severe hypoglycemia with this drug than with other oral agents, with prolonged action.	7

GENERIC NAME	BRAND NAME	ASSOCIATED DNI	REFERENCE
Tolbutamide (Antidiabetic)	**Orinase** (Upjohn)	Risk of hypoglycemia less than for chlorpropamide.	
		May give false-positive test for albumin in urine.	8
Acetohexamide (Antidiabetic)	**Dymelor** (Lilly)	Mildly diuretic; need to ensure adequate fluid intake.	9
Glyburide (Antidiabetic)	**DiaBeta** (Hoescht-Roussel) **Micronase** (Upjohn)	Risk of severe hypoglycemia; see chlorpropamide.	
Glipizide (Antidiabetic)	**Glucotrol** (Roerig)	Short-acting drug. Beneficial DNI includes control of early postprandial hyperglycemia.	10
Tolazamide (Antidiabetic)	**Tolinase** (Upjohn)	This drug, like other oral agents, is bound to plasma proteins. In protein-energy malnutrition (PEM) with hypoalbuminemia, more drug is freed to increase hypoglycemic effect.	11

Risk factors for hypoglycemia with oral antidiabetic agents

1. Due to the drug regimen: Hypoglycemia is most likely with the use of long-acting oral antidiabetic agents, such as chlorpropamide.

2. Due to the diet regimen: Include an irregular diet, days without eating, and intake of alcoholic beverages.
3. Due to disease: Patients with diseases from which there are therapeutic indications for drugs that reduce blood sugar are at greater risk for hypoglycemia. This includes sulfa drugs given for infection and high doses of aspirin and related drugs given for arthritis treatment.

Risk factors for hyperglycemia in diabetics on therapy related to drug regimen

Concurrent intake of diabetogenic drugs including corticosteroids and thiazide diuretics.

1. Due to the diet regimen: Noncompliance with diabetic diet.
2. Due to disease: Presence of infection.

IV.2.

THYROTOXICOSIS AND MYXEDEMA

A. *Drugs used in primary disease control*

GENERIC NAME	BRAND NAME	ASSOCIATED DNI	REFERENCE
Levothyroxine (Thyroid hormone)	**Synthroid** (Flint)	Anticoagulant effects of warfarin may be potentiated.	1
Propylthiouracil (Antithyroid)	**Propylthiouracil**	Anticoagulant effects of warfarin may be potentiated.	2
		Loss of taste may be a problem.	2
		Weight gain may be due to edema and renal complications.	

Risk factors for hemorrhage in patients on thyroid medications

1. Related to drug regimen: Intake of anticoagulants and lack of monitoring of prothrombin time.
2. Related to diet regimen: A diet low in vitamin K.
3. Related to disease: Risk is related to the presence of other diseases associated with the hemorrhagic state.

SECTION IV.1 REFERENCES

1. Muhlhauser I, Berger M, Sonnenberg G, Koch J, Jorgens V, Schernhaner G, Scholz V. Incidence and management of severe hypoglycaemia in 434 adults with insulin-dependent diabetes mellitus. *Diabetes Care.* 1985;8:268–273.
2. Woods SC, Porte D Jr. Insulin and the set point regulation of body weight. In: Novin D, Wyrwicka W, Bray G, eds. *Hunger: Basic Mechanisms and Clinical Applications.* New York: Raven Press; 1976:273–295.
3. Ferner RE, Neil HAW. Sulfonylureas and hypoglycaemia. *Br Med J.* 1988; 296:949–950.
4. Groop L, Koskimies S, Tolppanen E-M. Characterization of patients with chlorpropamide-alcohol flush. *Acta Med Scand.* 1984;215:141–149.
5. Luethi A, Studer H. Antidiuretic action of chlorpropamide and tolbutamide. Minn Med. 1969;52:33–35.
6. Isacson D, Stalhammar J. Prescription drug use among diabetics: a population study. *J Chron Dis.* 1987;40:651–660.
7. Pohl JEF, Hormones. In: *Geriatric Pharmacology and Therapeutics.* Brocklehurst JC, ed. Oxford, London: Blackwell Sci Pub; 1984:253.
8. *Facts and Comparisons.* 1988:382–386.
9. *Facts and Comparisons.* 1988:387.
10. Groop L, Melander A, Groop P-H, Ratheiser K, Simonson DC, DeFronzo RA. Different effects of glyburide and glipizide on insulin secretion and hepatic glucose production in normal and NIDDM subjects. *Diabetes.* 1987; 36:1320-1328.
11. Krishnaswamy K. Effects of malnutrition on drug metabolism and toxicity in humans. In: *Nutritional Toxicology.* Vol 2. Hathcock, JN, ed. New York: Academic Press; 1987:105–128.

SECTION IV.2 REFERENCES

1. Hansten PD. *Drug Interactions.* Philadelphia: Lea and Febiger; 1985:98–99.
2. *Facts and Comparisons.* 1988:409.

Section

V

Musculoskeletal Disease

SECTION V MUSCULOSKELETAL DISEASE

V.1. RHEUMATOID ARTHRITIS

A. *Drugs used in primary disease control*

GENERIC NAME	BRAND NAME	ASSOCIATED DNI	REFERENCE
Penicillamine (Anti-inflammatory)	**Cuprimine** (MSD) **Depen** (Wallace)	May cause zinc deficiency with distortion of taste, anorexia, and weight loss.	1
		Vitamin B_6 antagonist. A daily supplement (25 mg) of B_6 is advised.	2
Gold sodium thiomalate (Anti-inflammatory)	**Myochrysine**	Nephrotoxic, may cause nephrosis and protein deficiency.	3
Prednisone (Anti-inflammatory)		High risk of osteoporosis. See further information under Section II.1.	4
Methotrexate (Anti-inflammatory)	**Rheumatrex** (Lederle)	Stomatitis, enteritis, and leukopenia occur due to acute antifolate effects.	5

GENERIC NAME	BRAND NAME	ASSOCIATED DNI	REFERENCE
		Malabsorption, hepatic toxicity and megaloblastic anemia occur due to chronic antifolate effects.	6
		Teratogenic.	7
		1 mg folic acid/day can reduce adverse GI effects with low-dose therapy. See Section VIII.	8

B. ***Drugs used in control of secondary problems*** (includes control of joint pain and swelling)

GENERIC NAME	BRAND NAME	ASSOCIATED DNI	REFERENCE
Aspirin (Anti-inflammatory)	**Empirin** (B-W)	May cause anemia due to GI blood loss.	9
	Ecotrin (Smith)	Can cause a reduction in serum folate.	10
		Increases vitamin & loss in urine.	

V.2.
OSTEOARTHRITIS

A. *Drugs used in primary disease control*

GENERIC NAME	BRAND NAME	ASSOCIATED DNI	REFERENCE
Diflunisal (NSAID)*	**Dolobid** (MSD)	NSAIDs drugs impose a risk of GI blood loss leading to anemia.	1
Fenoprofen (NSAID)	**Nalfon** (Dista)	NSAIDs can induce fluid retention and weight gain.	2
Indomethacin (NSAID)	**Indocin** (MSD)	NSAIDs impose risk of hyperkalemia, which is most likely in those with renal disease, those taking potassium supplements, or those using salt substitutes or taking potassium-sparing diuretics.	3
Ketoprofen (NSAID)	**Orudis** (Wyeth)		
Meclofenamate (NSAID)	**Meclomen** (Parke Davis)		
Naproxen (NSAID)	**Anaprox** (Syntex) **Naprosyn** (Syntex)		
Piroxicam (NSAID)	**Feldene** (Pfizer)		

GENERIC NAME	BRAND NAME	ASSOCIATED DNI	REFERENCE
Sulindac (NSAID)	**Clinoril** (MSD)	NSAIDs such as Sulindac may contain the food dye tartrazine, which is a common cause of urticaria (hives).	4
Tolmetin (NSAID)	**Tolectin** (McNeil)		5

NOTE: These DNIs, as well as indigestion and risk of peptic ulcer, may be associated with intake of any NSAID (including ibuprofen).

For further information on risk of the different drugs within the group, see refs 1-5.

*NSAID = Nonsteroidal antiinflammatory drug.

V.3.
GOUT

A. *Drugs used in primary disease control*

GENERIC NAME	BRAND NAME	ASSOCIATED DNI	REFERENCE
Colchicine (Antigout)	**Colchicine** (Lilly) **ColBenemid** (MSD)	Can cause malabsorption and weight loss, but rarely a serious problem because of short duration of drug use.	1
Allopurinol (Antigout)	**Zyloprim** (Burroughs-Wellcome) **Lopurin** (Boots)	Prolongs the action of anticoagulants such as warfarin, which are vitamin K antagonists.	2
		Drug clearance rate is slowed by low-protein diet.	3

GENERIC NAME	BRAND NAME	ASSOCIATED DNI	REFERENCE
		Control of gout with allopurinol may be reduced by concurrent intake of thiazides.	4

B. *Drugs used to treat secondary problems*

GENERIC NAME	BRAND NAME	ASSOCIATED DNI	REFERENCE
Probenecid (Uricosuric)	**Benemid** (MSD)	If given with a diet that is associated with acid urine, the risk of kidney stones is increased. Diets producing acid urine are high in purines and protein.	5

Risk factors for drug-nutrient interactions in patients with arthritis

1. Risk factors for zinc deficiency in patients with rheumatoid arthritis who are receiving penicillamine include concurrent high intake of alcoholic beverage and previous use of nephrotoxic drugs (eg, gold salts).
2. Risk factors for iron deficiency anemia in patients on nonsteroidal antiinflammatory drugs include intake of the drug by patients with peptic ulcers and by those whose dietary intake of iron is less than the RDA.
3. Risk factors for hyperkalemia in patients on NSAIDs is increased in patients with renal disease; in those who take potassium-sparing diuretics, in those taking potassium supplements, and in those using potassium-containing salt substitutes.

4. Risk factors for malabsorption in patients with gout who are taking colchicine include prolonged intake of the drug, previous evidence of malabsorption due to gluten-sensitive enteropathy, and high intake of alcohol, which can also reduce nutrient absorption.

SECTION V.1 REFERENCES

1. Lyle WH. Penicillamine and zinc. *Lancet.* 1974;2:1140.
2. Rumsby PC, Shepherd DM. The effect of penicillamine on vitamin B_6 function in man. *Biochem Pharmacol.* 1981;30:3051–3053.
3. *Facts and Comparisons.* 1988:949.
4. Leonards JH, Levy G. Gastrointestinal blood loss during prolonged aspirin administration. *N Engl J Med.* 1975;289:1020–1022.
5. Sullivan RD, Miller E, Sikes MP. Antimetabolite-metabolite combination cancer chemotherapy: effects of intra-arterial methotrexateintramuscular citrovorum factor therapy in human cancer. *Cancer.* 1959;12:1248–1262.
6. Nohlaard C, Rubio CA, Kock Y, Hammar H. Liver fibrosis is quantified in methotrexate-treated patients with psoriasis. *Am Acad Dermatol.* 1993;28: 40–45.
7. Schorr EB, Steinbach HL. Aminopterin-induced fetal malformation: survival of infant after attempted abortion. *Am J Dis Child.* 1968;115:477–482.
8. Morgan SL, Baggott JE, Vaugn WH, Young PK, Austin JV, Krumdieck CL, Alarcon GS. The effect of folic acid supplementation on the toxicity of low-dose methotrexate in patients with rheumatoid arthritis. *Arthrit Rheum.* 1990; 33:9–18.
9. Lawrence VA, Loewenstein JE, Eichner ER. Aspirin and folate binding: in vivo and in vitro studies of serum binding and urinary excretion of endogenous folate. *J Lab Clin Med.* 1984;103:944–948.
10. Roe DA. *Drug-Induced Nutritional Deficiencies.* 2nd ed. Westport, Conn: AVI Publ Co; 1985:179–180.

SECTION V.2 REFERENCES

1. Carson JL, Strom BL, Soper KA, West SL, Lee Morse M. The association of non-steroidal anti-inflammatory drugs with upper gastrointestinal tract bleeding. *Arch Intern Med.* 1987;147:85–88.
2. Agnholt J, Andreasen F. The effect of ibuprofen therapy on water and electrolyte balance. *Acta Med Scand.* 1982;212:65–69.
3. Lamy PP. Renal effects of non-steroidal anti-inflammatory drugs. Heightened risk to the elderly? *J Am Geriatr Soc.* 1986;34:361–365.
4. Roe DA. *Diet and Drug Interactions.* New York: Van Nostrand Reinhold; 1988:73–74.
5. *USPDI.* 11th ed. 1991:450–499.

SECTION V.3 REFERENCES

1. Roe DA. *Drug-Induced Nutritional Deficiencies.* 1985:159–160.
2. Hansten PD. *Drug Interactions.* 5th ed. Philadelphia: Lea and Febiger; 1985: 67.
3. Park GD, Berlinger WG, Spector R, Kitt TM, Tsalikian E. Sustained reductions in oxypurinol renal clearance during a restricted diet. *Clin Pharmacol Ther.* 1987;41:616–621.
4. *USPDI.* Vol I.A. 1988:963.
5. Grahame-Smith DG, Aronson JK. *Oxford Textbook of Clinical Pharmacology and Drug Therapy.* Oxford, New York: Oxford Univ Press; 1984:490.

Section
VI
Neuropsychiatric Disease

SECTION
VI NEUROPSYCHIATRIC DISEASE

VI.I. SEIZURE DISORDERS

A. *Drugs used in primary disease control*

GENERIC NAME	BRAND NAME	ASSOCIATED DNI	REFERENCE
Phenytoin (Anticonvulsant)	**Dilantin** (Parke-Davis)	Phenytoin can induce folate deficiency with development of megaloblastic anemia.	1
		Vitamin D deficiency may develop in children and adults on long-term intake of this drug.	2
		Vitamin K deficiency with bleeding may develop, especially in infants of mothers who have been on the drug.	3

GENERIC NAME	BRAND NAME	ASSOCIATED DNI	REFERENCE
		Phenytoin can potentiate effect of anticoagulants.	4
		High intake of folic acid (>5 mg/day) can interfere with seizure control.	5
		Incompatibility of the drug with formula foods has been reported; this can reduce drug absorption and seizure control. Nasogastric tube blockage can occur if the drug is given during continuous formula infusion.	6
		Milk consumption at the time phenytoin is given will not significantly reduce drug uptake.	7
		Morbidly obese patients require high loading doses of phenytoin to achieve therapeutic drug concentrations.	8
Phenobarbital (Anticonvulsant)	**Phenobarbital** (various)	Depressant effects of this drug enhanced by alcohol. For anti-vitamin effects, see Phenytoin.	9

GENERIC NAME	BRAND NAME	ASSOCIATED DNI	REFERENCE
Primidone (Anticonvulsant)	**Mysoline** (Ayerst)	Megaloblastic anemia due to folate depletion can occur, as with phenytoin.	10
Paramethadione (Anticonvulsant)	**Paradione** (Abbott)	Contains tartrazine, which can cause hives or asthma.	11
Valproic acid (Anticonvulsant)	**Depakene** (Abbott)	Carnitine deficiency has been reported with hyperammonemia. Coma may occur with this complication.	12
		Coagulation defects may occur with risk of bleeding & anemia.	13
		Valproic acid passes into breast milk, 1-10% of serum concentration.	14
		Valproic acid is teratogenic; associated neural tube defects may be folate-related.	15
Carbamazepine (Anticonvulsant)	**Tegretol** (Geigy)	May cause unpleasant taste and anorexia.	16
		Soreness of the mouth; hence, failure to eat may indicate aplastic anemia.	17

GENERIC NAME	BRAND NAME	ASSOCIATED DNI	REFERENCE
		Maintenance dose of carbamazepine should be reduced and dose interval prolonged in obese subjects. Clearance of this drug increases with marked weight reduction.	18

Risk factors related to adverse outcomes of drug-nutrient interactions for patients with seizure disorders

1. Risk factors for folate deficiency in patients with seizure disorders receiving phenytoin include concurrent intake of other anticonvulsants including phenobarbital (which also can induce folate deficiency), low intake of dietary folate sources, and a history of malabsorption.
2. Risk factors for osteomalacia or rickets in patients on phenytoin include institutionalization, being homebound, having a zero or very low milk intake, and concurrently taking anticonvulsant drugs that can cause vitamin D deficiency, including phenobarbital.
3. Risk factors for vitamin K deficiency with bleeding exist in infants of mothers who have taken phenytoin with or without phenobarbital through pregnancy, particularly in those mothers who have not received vitamin K supplements during the third trimester.
4. Risk of rickets or osteomalacia is greatest when there is no sun or UV exposure and no intake of milk. Moderate vitamin D supplements (1000-2000 iu/day) will prevent risk.
5. The risk of neural tube defects (NTD) in pregnant women on valproic acid is higher in those with a previous history of having an infant with NTD and folate depletion.

VI.2.

PARKINSON'S DISEASE

A. *Drugs used in primary disease control*

GENERIC NAME	BRAND NAME	ASSOCIATED DNI	REFERENCE
Levodopa (Anti-Parkinson)	**Dopar** (Norwich Eaton)	Vitamin products containing B_6 should be avoided; they may interfere with disease control.	1
		The brand cited contains tartrazine and should therefore be avoided by those having reactions to tartrazine in food.	2
		Should be taken with food to avoid irritation, but not with meat, other high-protein food or protein hydrolysates, because amino acids can impair drug absorption.	3
		Anorexia is a problem in 50% of patients on this drug.	4

GENERIC NAME	BRAND NAME	ASSOCIATED DNI	REFERENCE
		Use of this drug with MAOI drugs and food amine sources (beans or cheese) is contraindicated, due to the risk of tyramine reaction, causing acute hypertension.	5
		Risk of vitamin B_6 deficiency with high dosage.	6
		Levodopa may cause hypokalemia.	7
		May interfere with urine tests for sugar and ketones.	8
Carbidopa + Levodopa (Anti-Parkinson)	**Sinemet** (MSD)	See Levodopa; but risk of vitamin B_6 deficiency is less than with levodopa alone.	9

B. *Drugs used to treat secondary problems*

GENERIC NAME	BRAND NAME	ASSOCIATED DNI	REFERENCE
Amantadine (Dopaminergic)	**Symmetrel** (DuPont)	Dry mouth may be a problem; also constipation.	10
Benztropine (Anticho-linergic)	**Cogentin** (MSD)	See amantadine.	
Bromocriptine (Dopamine receptor agonist)	**Parlodel** (Sandoz)	Nausea & anorexia may occur.	11

Risk factors

Risk of hypokalemia in Parkinson's disease patients on preparations containing Levodopa is greatest if potassium-losing diuretics are being taken concurrently and/or if laxatives are being taken.

Risk factors for dry mouth and anorexia in patients taking anticholinergic drugs for Parkinson's disease include advanced age, high drug dose and Sjogren's disease. In addition, patients should avoid taking anticholinergic, antispasmodic drugs for other problems (eg, irritable bowel syndrome), such as Donnatal (Robins), concurrently with amantadine or anticholinergic drugs (ref 12).

VI.3.
MANIC-DEPRESSIVE PSYCHOSIS AND OTHER DEPRESSIVE STATES

A. *Drugs used in primary disease control*

GENERIC NAME	BRAND NAME	ASSOCIATED DNI	REFERENCE
Lithium (Antimania)	**Eskalith** (SKF) **Cibalith-S** (Ciba)	Reduction in sodium or diuretic intake can induce lithium toxicity with nausea, weight gain due to edema, thirst, confusion, and coma.	1
		Increases in sodium intake will decrease the effectiveness of the drug.	2
		Weight gain in those on this drug may be due to increases in appetite and food intake.	3
Phenelzine (MAOI-antidepressant)	**Nardil** (Parke-Davis)	Tyramine reactions may occur with acute hypertension if aged cheese or other high-tyramine foods are consumed. Other MAOI antidepressants (eg, Tranyl cypromine) carry the same risk.	4

GENERIC NAME	BRAND NAME	ASSOCIATED DNI	REFERENCE
Imipramine (Antidepressant)	**Tofranil** (Geigy)	May interfere with the biochemical assessment of riboflavin status or induce riboflavin depletion. Other tricyclic antidepressants carry the same nutritional risk.	5
		Appetite may be increased in some patients on tricyclic antidepressants.	6

B. ***Drugs used to treat secondary problems (sedatives, stimulants, and drugs to treat insomnia)***

GENERIC NAME	BRAND NAME	ASSOCIATED DNI	REFERENCE
Lorazepam (Antianxiety)	**Ativan** (Wyeth)	Drowsiness may interfere with food intake.	7
Flurazepam (Antiinsomnia)	**Dalmane** (Roche)	See Lorazepam.	
Temazepam (Antiinsomnia)	**Restoril** (Sandoz)	See Lorazepam.	
Methylphenidate (Stimulant)	**Ritalin** (Ciba)	When given to children, may retard growth due to anorexia and low food intake, or may result in weight loss in hyperactive children.	8

Risk factors

1. Diet-related risk of lithium toxicity includes a sudden switch to a low-sodium conventional diet or a low-sodium formula diet.
2. Risk of a tyramine reaction in patients on MAOI antidepressants is greatest when aged cheese or dishes containing aged cheese are eaten at the time of drug intake.

VI.4.

DEMENTIAS AND PARANOID STATES

A. *Drugs of proven benefit in control of behavior*

GENERIC NAME	BRAND NAME	ASSOCIATED DNI	REFERENCE
Chlorpromazine (Antipsychotic)	**Thorazine** (SKF)	Phenothiazines (including this drug) increase appetite, and if the patient has free access to food, this may lead to a food energy intake in excess of need, resulting in obesity.	1
		Fluid retention with resultant weight gain & hyponatremia with associated confusion may occur in those who take this drug daily.	2

GENERIC NAME	BRAND NAME	ASSOCIATED DNI	REFERENCE
		This phenothiazine may interfere with the biochemical assessment of riboflavin status & may also induce riboflavin depletion.	3
Thioridazine (Antipsychotic)	**Mellaril** (Sandoz)	See Chlorpromazine.	
		Liquid preparations are incompatible with enteral formulas. Can lead to blockage of nasogastric tubes if given during formula infusion.	4
Perphenazine (Antipsychotic)	**Trilafon** (Schering)	See Chlorpromazine.	
Fluphenazine (Antipsychotic)	**Prolixin** (Princeton)	See Chlorpromazine.	
Thiothixene (Antipsychotic)	**Navane** (Roerig)	See Chlorpromazine.	
Prochlorperazine (Antiemetic/ antipsychotic)	**Compazine** (SKF)	Used to control nausea; may be given orally or rectally.	5
Haloperidol (Antiemetic/ antipsychotic)	**Haldol** (McNeil)	Constipation may be a problem. Contains tartrazine; dry mouth may occur.	6

B. ***Drugs employed to alleviate symptoms (drugs used as adjuncts to major antipsychotic drugs and those purported to improve cerebral circulation)***

GENERIC NAME	BRAND NAME	ASSOCIATED DNI	REFERENCE
Diazepam (Antianxiety)	**Valium** (Roche)	Dry mouth may reduce food intake if given in high doses.	7
Pentoxifylline (Anti-TIA)	**Trental** (Hoescht-Roussel)	Anorexia & nausea may reduce food intake.	8

Risk factors

Risk of excessive weight gain in patients on phenothiazine tranquilizers is greatest if there is multiple access to snack foods and intake of a regular diet. The risk is greater for ambulatory patients.

VI.5.
ALCOHOLISM

A. ***Drugs used in primary disease control***

GENERIC NAME	BRAND NAME	ASSOCIATED DNI	REFERENCE
Disulfiram (Alcohol aversion drug)	**Antabuse** (Ayerst)	Intended effect is disulfiram reaction (headache, nausea, vomiting, and chest pain) when alcohol is consumed.	1

B. *Drugs used in the control of secondary problems (includes drugs used to prevent liver failure)*

GENERIC NAME	BRAND NAME	ASSOCIATED DNI	REFERENCE
Lactulose (Laxative/ anti-liver failure)	**Cephulac** (Merrell Dow)	Intended effect is reduction of blood ammonia levels.	2

Risk factors

Risk of disulfiram reactions in alcoholics on disulfiram (Antabuse) is greatest for those who mistakenly believe that if they stop the drug, they can immediately drink alcohol without inducing an adverse reaction.

SECTION VI.I REFERENCES

1. Reynolds EH, Milner G, Matthews DM, Chanarin I. Anticonvulsant therapy, megaloblastic haemopoiesis and folic acid metabolism. *Quart J Med.* 1966; 35:521–537.
2. Hahn TJ, Halstead LR. Anticonvulsant drug-induced osteomalacia: alterations in mineral metabolism and response to vitamin D_3 administration. *Calcif Tiss Internat.* 1979;27:13–18.
3. Mountain KR, Hirsch J, Gallus AS. Neonatal coagulation defect due to anticonvulsant drug treatment in pregnancy. *Lancet.* 1970;1:265–268.
4. Hansten PD. *Drug Interactions.* 5th ed. Philadelphia: Lea & Febiger; 1985: 92.
5. Mattson RH, Gallagher BB, Reynolds EN, Glass D. Folate therapy in epilepsy: a controlled study. *Arch Neurol.* 1973;29:78–81.
6. Bauer LA. Interference of oral phenytoin absorption by continuous nasogastric feedings. *Neurology.* 1982;32:570–572.
7. Dotson R, Dickinson L, Hang N, Dashieff R. Effect of simultaneously ingested milk on phenytoin bioavailability. *Neurology.* 1985;35:1526–1527.
8. Abernethy DR, Greenblatt DJ. Phenytoin disposition in obesity: determination of the loading dose. *Arch Neurol.* 1985;42:468–471.
9. Seitz HK. Alcohol effects on drug-nutrient interactions. *Drug-Nutr Interact.* 1985;4:143–163.
10. Chanarin I. *The Megaloblastic Anaemias.* Oxford: Blackwell Sci Publ; 1969: 830–843.
11. *Facts and Comparisons.* 1988:1152.
12. Ohtani Y, Endo F, Matsuda I. Carnitine deficiency and hyperammonemia associated with valproic acid therapy. *J Pediatr.* 1982;101:782–785.
13. Hyams DE. Central nervous system: antiParkinsonism and antiepileptic drugs. In: Brocklehurst JC, ed. *Geriatric Pharmacology and Therapeutics.* London: Blackwell Sci Publ; 1984:174.

14. Janas LM, Picciano MF. Human milk: a portal of drugs from mother to infant. In: Roe DA, Campbell, TC, eds. *Drugs and Nutrients: The Interactive Effects.* New York: Marcel Dekker; 1984:344.
15. Wegner C, Nau H. Alteration of embryonic folate metabolism by valproic acid during organogenesis. *Neurology.* 1992;42(suppl. 5):17–24.
16. Bork K. *Cutaneous Side Effects of Drugs.* Philadelphia: WB Saunders Co; 1988:309.
17. *Drug Facts and Comparisons.* 1992:1392-1396.
18. Caraco Y, Zylber-Katz E, Berry EM, Levy M. Significant weight reduction in obese subjects enhances carbamazepine elimination. *Clin Pharmacol Ther.* 1992;51:501–506.

SECTION VI.2. REFERENCES

1. Duvoisin RC, Yahr MD, Cote LD. Reversal of ''dopa effect'' in Parkinsonism by pyridoxine. *Trans Am Neurol Assoc.* 1969;94:81-84.
2. Roe DA. *Diet and Drug Interactions.* New York: Van Nostrand Reinhold; 1988:73-74.
3. Roe DA. *Drug-Induced Nutritional Deficiencies.* 2nd ed. New York: AVI Publ Co; 1985:293-299.
4. MacLennan WJ, Shepherd AN, Stevenson IH. *The Elderly.* New York: Springer Verlag; 1984:134.
5. *Facts and Comparisons.* 1988:1226-1228.
6. Golden RL, Mortati FS, Schroeter GA. Levodopa, pyridoxine and the burning feet syndrome. *JAMA.* 1970;213:628.
7. Granerus AK, Jagenburg R, Svanborg A. Kaliuretic effects of L-dopa treatment in Parkinsonian patients. *Acta Med Scand.* 1981;647(suppl):75-85.
8. Hansten PD. *Drug Interactions.* 2nd ed. 1971:419.
9. Parkes JD. Adverse effects of antiparkinsonian drugs. *Drugs.* 1981;21:341-353.
10. Hyams DE. Central nervous system, antiparkinsonism and antiepileptic drugs: use of drugs in stroke. In: *Geriatric Pharmacology and Therapeutics.* 1984:170-171.
11. *Fact and Comparisons.* 1988:1232.

SECTION VI.3 REFERENCES

1. Fieve RR. *The Practical Uses of Lithium.* London: Norgine Ltd.; 1979:10-11.
2. Hyams DE. Central nervous system, antidepressants. In: *Geriatric Pharmacology and Therapeutics.* 1984:149-150.
3. Vendsborg PB, Bech P, Rafaelsen OJ. Lithium treatment and weight gain. *Acta Psychiatr Scand.* 1976;53:139-147.
4. Blackwell B, Mabbitt LA. Tyramine in cheese related to hypertensive crises after monoamine oxidase inhibition. *Lancet.* 1965;1:940-943.

5. Pinto JT, Rivlin RS. Drugs that promote renal excretion of riboflavin. *Drug-Nutrient Interact.* 1987;5:143-151.
6. Levitsky DA. Drugs, appetite and body weight. In: *Drugs and Nutrients: The Interactive Effects.* 1984:390-391.
7. *Facts and Comparisons.* 1988:996.
8. Safer D, Allen R, Barr E. Depression of growth in hyperactive children on stimulant drugs. *N Engl J Med.* 1972;287:217-220.

SECTION VI.4 REFERENCES

1. Doss FW. The effect of antipsychotic drugs on appetite: a retrospective review. *J Clin Psychiatr.* 1979;40:528-530.
2. Shah DK, Wig NN, Chaudhury RR. Antidiuretic hormone levels in patients with weight gain after chlorpromazine therapy. *Indian J Med Res.* 1973;61: 771-776.
3. Pelliccione N, Pinto J, Huang YP, Rivlin RS. Acceleration of development of riboflavin deficiency by treatment with chlor- promazine. *Biochem Pharmacol.* 1983;32:2949-2953.
4. Cutie AJ, Altman E, Lenkel L. Compatibility of enteral products with commonly employed drug additives. JPEN. 1983;7:176-179.
5. *Facts and Comparisons.* 1988:972.
6. Hamdy RC. *Geriatric Nutrition.* Philadelphia: Balliere Tindall; 1984:158-160.
7. Powers DE, Moore AO. *Food Medication Interactions.* 5th ed. Phoenix: F-MI Publ; 1986:65.
8. *Facts and Comparisons.* 1988:215.

SECTION VI.5 REFERENCES

1. Faiman MD. Biochemical pharmacology of disulfiram. In: Majchrowicz E, Noble EP, eds. *Biochemistry and Pharmacology of Ethanol.* Vol 2. New York: Plenum Press; 1979:325-348.
2. Roe DA. *Alcohol and the Diet.* Westport, Conn: AVI Publ Co; 1979:198.

Section

VII

Dermatological Disease

SECTION

VII DERMATOLOGICAL DISEASE

VII.1. ACNE

A. *Drugs used in primary disease control*

GENERIC NAME	BRAND NAME	ASSOCIATED DNI	REFERENCE
Isotretinoin (Antiacne)	**Accutane** (Roche)	This drug is a structural analogue of vitamin A. Adverse effects resemble those associated with vitamin A overload.	1
		Skeletal changes with bony spurs similar to those seen in vitamin A toxicity may occur if treatment for acne or for another dermatosis that is responsive to the drug is longer than 3 months, or if the drug level is >1 mg/kg.	2

GENERIC NAME	BRAND NAME	ASSOCIATED DNI	REFERENCE
		Isotretinoin can cause increases in both plasma triglyceride and plasma cholesterol.	3
		This drug is teratogenic.	4
		The major risk of elevated triglyceride levels is acute pancreatitis.	5
		Absorption of this drug is increased by food.	6
Tetracycline (Antiacne)	**Achromycin V** (Lederle) **Panmycin** (Upjohn) **Robitet** (Robins) **Sumycin** (Squibb)	See Section II.2.A.	

NOTE: Whenever possible doxycycline, rather than tetracycline, should be used for treatment of adolescent acne. Doxycycline does not form insoluble complexes with calcium in foods, so there is no need to limit milk intake.

*Risk factors for retinoid toxicity**

1. Related to drug regimen: Intake of more than 1 mg/kg isotretinoin is associated with a significantly increased risk of these side effects.
2. Related to diet: Risk of hypercholesterolemia and hypertriglyceridemia in patients on isotretinoin or on etretinate is increased by intake of a high-cholesterol diet, by high intake of vitamin A supplements, and by high intake of alcoholic beverages. If retinoid-associated hyperlipidemia does not respond to reduction in fat and cholesterol intake or dose reduction, the drug should be discontinued (see ref 10).

3. Related to disease: Risk of hepatic damage due to retinoids is increased by the presence of alcoholic hepatitis, cirrhosis, viral hepatitis, or hepatitis due to other drugs.

*These risk factors apply to other synthetic retinoids, eg, etretinate.

VII.2.
PSORIASIS

GENERIC NAME	BRAND NAME	ASSOCIATED DNI	REFERENCE
Etretinate (Antipsoriatic)	**Tegison** (Roche)	Milk consumed with the drug increases absorption.	7
		Certain DNI are similar to isotretinoin.	8
		GI effects not found with isotretinoin, but common effects with this drug include anorexia, taste perversion, oral ulcers, and diarrhea.	9
Methoxsalen (Antipsoriatic)	**Oxsoralen** (Elder)	May cause GI irritation. Drug should be taken with milk.	10

GENERIC NAME	BRAND NAME	ASSOCIATED DNI	REFERENCE
Cyclosporine (Antipsoriatic)	**Sandimmune** (Sandoz)	Food promotes oral absorption. Main use of drug is to prevent graft rejection. Food promotes clearance when the drug is given iv. High-fat meals given with oral drug doses promote drug absorption more than low-fat meals.	11
		Nephrotoxic.	12
		May increase BP, cholesterol level, and magnesium loss.	13
		Frequently elevates uric acid levels, and may precipitate gout.	14,15

SECTION VII. REFERENCES

1. van der Meeren HLM, van der Schroeff JG, Schijnen T, van Duren JA, van der Dries HAC, van Voorst Vader PC. Dose-response relationships in isotretinoin therapy in conglobate acne. *Dermatologica.* 1983;167:299-303.
2. Ellis CN, Pennes DR, Hermann RC, Blauvelt BS, Martel W, Voorhees JJ. Long-term radiographic follow-up after isotretinoin therapy. *J Am Acad Dermatol.* 1988;18:1252-1261.
3. Bershad S, Rubinstein A, Paterniti JR, Le NA, Poliak SC, Heller B, Ginsburg HN, Fleischmajer R, Virgil Brown W. Changes in plasma lipids and lipoproteins during isotretinoin acne therapy. *N Engl J Med.* 1985;313:981-985.
4. Lammer EJ, Chen DT, Hoar RM, Agnish ND, Benke PJ, Braun JT, Curry CJ, Fernhoff PM, Grix AW, Lott IT, Richard JM, Sun SC. Retinoic acid embryopathy. *N Engl J Med.* 1985;313:837-841.

5. Zech LA, Gross ED, Perck GL, Bryan Brewer H. Changes in plasma cholesterol and triglyceride levels after treatment with oral isotretinoin: prospective study. *Arch Dermatol.* 1983;119:987-993.
6. Colburn WA, Gibson DM, Wiens RE, Hanigan JJ. Food increases the bioavailability of isotretinoin. *J Clin Pharmacol.* 1983;23:534-539.
7. *Drug Facts and Comparisons.* 1992:2188-2190.
8. Ellis CN, Voorhees JJ. Etretinate therapy. *J Am Acad Dermatol.* 1987;16: 267-291.
9. Lowe NJ, Lazarus V, Matt L. Systemic retinoid therapy for psoriasis. *J Am Acad Dermatol.* 1988;19:186-191.
10. Saurat JR. Side effects of systemic retinoids and their clinical management. *J Am Acad Dermatol.* 1992;27:523-528.
11. *Drug Facts and Comparisons.* 1992:2608-2609.
12. Gupta SK, Mamfro RC, Tomlanovich SJ, Gambertoglio JG, Garavoy MR, Benet LZ. Effect of food on the pharmacokinetics of cyclosporine in healthy subjects following oral and intravenous administration. *J Clin Pharmacol.* 1990;30:643-653.
13. *Drug Facts and Comparisons.* 1992:2592-2596.
14. De Rie MA, Meinardi MMHM, Bos JD. Analysis of side effects of medium- and low-dose cyclosporin maintenance therapy in psoriasis. *Br J Dermatol.* 1990;123:347-353.
15. Lin H-Y, Rocher LL, McQuillan MA, Schmaltz S, Pallela TD, Fox IN. Cyclosporine-induced hyperuricemia and gout. *N Engl J Med.* 1989;321: 287-292.

Section VIII
Neoplastic Disease

SECTION
VIII NEOPLASTIC DISEASE

Leukemia, Hodgkin's Disease, and Cancer

A. *Drugs used in primary disease control*

GENERIC NAME	BRAND NAME	ASSOCIATED DNI	REFERENCE
Procarbazine (Anti-Hodgkin's)	**Matulane** (Roche)	This drug is a monoamine oxidase inhibitor (MAOI). Acute hypertension can occur if the drug is given with tyramine-containing foods and/or other MAOI. The drug is also a vitamin B_6 antagonist.	1
		When used in Hodgkin's disease, may be with doxorubicin, cyclophosphamide, vincristine, & prednisone, which confers the risk of combined DNI of these drugs.	2

GENERIC NAME	BRAND NAME	ASSOCIATED DNI	REFERENCE
5-Fluorouracil (Antineoplastic)	**Adrucil** (Adria)	May cause anorexia, vomiting, & diarrhea. Stomatitis may limit food intake or may preclude intake of solid or dry foods during systemic therapy.	3
Bleomycin (Antineoplastic)	**Blenoxane** (Bristol Labs)	Pneumonitis & associated dyspnea may reduce food intake. May cause mouth ulcers and vomiting.	4
Carmustine (Antineoplastic)	**BiCNU** (Bristol Labs)	Nephrotoxic drug; can cause hypophosphatemia and glycosuria.	5
Cisplatin (Antineoplastic)	**Platinol** (Bristol Labs)	Drug is nephrotoxic; can cause magnesium depletion.	6
Cyclophosphamide (Antineoplastic)	**Cytoxan** (Mead-Johnson) **Neosar** (Adria)	Can cause vomiting and occasionally diarrhea.	3,7
Dactinomycin (Antineoplastic)	**Cosmegen** (MSD)	Nausea, vomiting, diarrhea & stomatitis are common side effects.	8
Doxorubicin (Antineoplastic)	**Adriamycin RDF** (Adria)	Cardiomyopathy is a major side effect. Vitamin E prevents the cardiotoxicity in rats, but not in humans.	9

GENERIC NAME	BRAND NAME	ASSOCIATED DNI	REFERENCE
Lomustine (Antineoplastic)	**CeeNu** (Bristol Labs)	Nausea and vomiting occur 3-6 hours after oral dose.	10
Methotrexate (Antineoplastic)	**Mexate** (Bristol Labs)	Stomatitis, anorexia, and diarrhea with malab-sorption are common with weight loss.	11
Trimetrexate (Antineoplastic)	**Trimetrexate** (Warner-Lambert)	This drug is a folate antagonist. Anemia with pancytopenia occurs. Folinic acid rescue necessary.	12
Vincristine (Antineoplastic)	**Oncovin** (Lilly)	Oral ulceration, nausea, vomiting & diarrhea may occur. Severe constipation is common.	13
		Risk of confusion & weakness due to hyponatremia. Side effects are similar with vinblastine.	14

B. *Drugs used as secondary agents to suppress tumor growth and drugs used to control pain*

GENERIC NAME	BRAND NAME	ASSOCIATED DNI	REFERENCE
Tamoxifen (Antiestrogenic)	**Nolvadex** (Stuart)	Hypercalcemia has been reported in patients with breast cancer and bone metastases treated with this drug.	15
Morphine (Narcotic analgesic)	**Astramorph PF** (Astra) **Duramorph** (Elkins-Sinn) **MS Contin** (Purdue-Frederick)	May increase anorexia and cause constipation.	16

Risk factors for GI side effects of antineoplastic agents

1. Related to drug regimen: High dosage of antineoplastic agents is associated with higher risk of these side effects. Ondansetron injections (Zofran, Cerenex Pharm) reduce the number of episodes of vomiting following cyclophosphamide therapy as compared with metoclopramide, which is alternatively employed to control vomiting (ref 17).
2. Related to diet: Risk of nausea and vomiting is related to large food intake within 3-6 hours of administration of the dose. This time interval varies for different drugs. Risk of acute folate deficiency in patients on methotrexate or trimetrexate includes lack of folinic acid rescue. Risk of a tyramine reaction in patients on procarbazine is related to ignorance by the patient and/or caregiver of the patient's need to exclude food sources of tyramine, (eg, cheese) from the diet during the treatment period.
3. Related to disease: Risk factors for magnesium depletion in cancer patients on cisplatin include previous renal impairment and all medical conditions associated with dehydration and hyper-

excretion of magnesium. This includes diseases requiring the use of loop diuretics.

SECTION VIII REFERENCES

1. Roe DA. *Diet and Drug Interactions.* New York: Van Nostrand Reinhold; 1988:63-64.
2. Weiss HB, Walker MD, Wiernik PH. Neurotoxicity of commonly used antineoplastic agents. *N Engl J Med.* 1974;291:75-81;127-133.
3. Carter SK. Nutritional problems associated with cancer chemotherapy. In: Newell GR, Ellison NM, eds. *Nutrition and Cancer: Etiology and Treatment.* New York: Raven Press; 1981:303-317.
4. Shils ME. Nutrition and diet in cancer. In: *Modern Nutrition in Health and Disease.* Philadelphia: Lea and Febiger; 1988:1412-1413.
5. Roe DA. *Drug-Induced Nutritional Deficiencies.* 2nd ed. New York: AVI Publ Co; 1985:301-306.
6. Schilsky R, Anderson T. Hypomagnesemia secondary to Cis-diammine-chlorplatinum II administration. *Ann Intern Med.* 1979;90:929-932.
7. Wiebe VJ, Benz CC, DeGregorio MW. Clinical pharmacokinetics of drugs used in the treatment of breast cancer. *Clin Pharmacokinet.* 1988;15:180-193.
8. Pratt WB, Ruddon RW. *The Anticancer Drugs.* New York: Oxford University Press; 1979:43-63.
9. Leghe SS, Wang YM, MacKay B, Ewer M, Hortobagyl GN, Benjamin RS, Ali MK. Clinical and pharmacologic investigation of the effects of alpha-tocopherol on adriamycin cardiotoxicity. *Ann NY Acad Sci.* 1982;393:411-418.
10. *Facts and Comparisons.* 1988:1985.
11. Jolivet J, Cowan KH, Curt GA, Clendeninn NJ, Chabner BA. The pharmacology and clinical use of methotrexate. *N Engl J Med.* 1983;309:1094-1104.
12. Balis FM, Patel R, Luks E, Doherty KM, Holcenberg JS, Tan C, Reaman GH, Belasco J, Ettinger LJ, Zimm S, Poplack DG. Pediatric phase I and pharmacokinetic study of trimetrexate. *Cancer Res.* 1987;47:4973-4976.
13. Sandler SG, Tubin W, Henderson ES. Vincristine-induced neuropathy: a clinical study of 50 leukemic patients. *Neurology.* 1969;19:367-374.
14. Oldham RK, Pomeroy TC. Vincristine-induced syndrome of inappropriate secretion of antidiuretic hormone. *South Med J.* 1972;65:1010.
15. *Facts and Comparisons.* 1988:2022-2023.
16. Grahame-Smith DG, Aronson JK. In: *Oxford Textbook of Clinical Pharmacology and Drug Therapy.* New York: Oxford University Press; 1984: 713-716.
17. *Drug Comparisons.* 1992:873-874.

Section IX
Infectious Disease

SECTION

IX

INFECTIOUS DISEASES (Viral, Protozoal, Fungal)

IX.1.

AIDS

A. *Drugs used in primary disease control*

GENERIC NAME	BRAND NAME	ASSOCIATED DNI	REFERENCE
Azidothymidine (AZT) (Antiviral)	**Retrovir** (Burroughs-Wellcome)	Drug-related anorexia, nausea and vomiting, and megaloblastic anemia may occur.	1

B. *Drugs used to control secondary protozoal and fungal infections (includes treatment of* Pneumocystis carinii *pneumonia and cryptococcal meningitis in AIDS patients)*

GENERIC NAME	BRAND NAME	ASSOCIATED DNI	REFERENCE
Pentamidine isethionate (Anti- and hypoglycemia, and protozoal agent)	**Pentam 300** (LyphoMed)	Metabolic side effects include hyperhypo-calcemia. Causes nausea, bad taste, & anorexia.	2,3
		Pentamidine can also cause folate deficiency.	4

GENERIC NAME	BRAND NAME	ASSOCIATED DNI	REFERENCE
Amphotericin B (Antifungal agent)	**Fungizone** (Squibb)	Used to treat cryptococcal meningitis. Frequently causes anorexia, nausea, vomiting, abdominal pain, diarrhea, weight loss and hypomagnesemia. Anemia and hypoanemia may occur. Nephrotoxic. Salt loading may prevent renal toxicity.	5,6
Fluconazole (Antifungal agent)	**Diflucan** (Roerig)	Used to treat cryptococcal meningitis. Nausea, vomiting, and diarrhea may occur.	7

Risk Factors

Risk factors for folate deficiency in a patient on pentamidine include low folate intake and malabsorption, which is common in AIDS patients.

C. ***Drugs used to treat secondary bacterial infections***

See Section II for drugs used to treat tuberculosis.

IX. 2.
GIARDIASIS

A. *Drugs used in primary disease control*

GENERIC NAME	BRAND NAME	ASSOCIATED DNI	REFERENCE
Metronidazole (Antiprotozoal agent)	**Flagyl** (Searle)	Alcohol should be avoided due to risk of disulfiram-like reaction, with nausea, headache, and vomiting.	8
		Disease causes lactose intolerance, which responds to treatment with this drug.	9

Risk Factors

Risk factors for disulfiram-like reactions in patients on metronidazole include the patient's being unaware of the need to exclude alcoholic beverages from the diet.

IX.3.
MALARIA

A. *Drugs used in primary disease control*

GENERIC NAME	BRAND NAME	ASSOCIATED DNI	REFERENCE
Pyrimethamine (Antiprotozoal)	**Daraprim** (Burroughs-Wellcome)	A folate antagonist; can cause megaloblastic anemia, which can be treated with folinic or folic acid.	10
Sulfadoxine + Pyrimethamine (Antiprotozoal)	**Fansidar** (Roche)	Antifolate effects of pyrimethamine impose risk of megaloblastic anemia. For low leukocyte or platelet count due to antifolate effects, present with overdosage, leucovorin (folinic acid), 5-15 mg im/day for 3 days, is recommended.	11
		GI symptoms may include stomatitis, which can limit food intake. Sulfa component of the drug combination can cause hypoglycemia in diabetics.	12

GENERIC NAME	BRAND NAME	ASSOCIATED DNI	REFERENCE
Chloroquine HCI (Antiprotozoal)	**Aralen HCI** (Winthrop-Breon)	Anemia due to hemolysis is a risk in those with glucose-6-phosphate dehydrogenase deficiency.	13

Risk Factors

Risk factors in patients taking pyrimethamine or drugs containing pyrimethamine and another agent include low dietary intake of folate and concurrent intake of other antifols, and malabsorption.

IX.4.
FUNGAL INFECTIONS

A. *Drugs used in primary disease control*

GENERIC NAME	BRAND NAME	ASSOCIATED DNI	REFERENCE
Griseofulvin (Antifungal)	**Fulvicin P/G** (Schering)	Best absorbed when taken with a meal containing fat, but ultra-micro-size formulations of drug are absorbed even without concurrent fat intake.	14
		May cause flush and/or headache if taken with alcohol.	15
Ketoconazole (Antifungal)	**Nizoral** (Janssen)	Nausea may occur, which can indicate hepatotoxicity.	16

		Should not be taken by women who are breast-feeding, due to risk of liver damage to the infant.	17
		Food decreases the absorption of the drug.	18
		May reduce serum cholesterol.	19
Amphotericin B (Antifungal)	**Fungizone** (Squibb)	Nephrotoxic. Can cause hypokalemia and hypomagnesemia.	20
		Weight loss is common with this drug.	21
		Normochromic, normocytic anemia may occur.	22

Risk factors for flush reactions

Risk factors for flush reactions in patients on griseofulvin include intake of alcoholic beverages with the drug.

SECTION IX REFERENCES

1. *Facts and Comparisons.* 1988:1561-1564.
2. *Facts and Comparisons.* 1988:1587-1588.
3. Hansten PD. *Drug Interactions.* Philadelphia: Lea and Febiger; 1973:328.
4. Weston KA, Perera DR, Schultz MG. Pentamidine isethionate in the treatment of *pneumocystis carinii* pneumonia. *Ann Intern Med.* 1970;73:695-702.
5. Tolins JP. Amphotericin versus fluconazole in cryptococcal meningitis. *N Engl J Med.* 1992;326:1567-1568.
6. Llanos A, Cieza J, Bernardo J, et al. *Kidney Int.* 1991;40:302-308.
7. Berry AJ, Rinaldi MO, Graybill GR. Use of high-dose fluconazole as salvage therapy for cryptococcal meningitis in patients with AIDS. *Antimicrob Agents Chemother.* 1993;36:690-692.

8. Seixas FA. Alcohol and its drug interactions. *Ann Intern Med.* 1975;83:86-92.
9. Scrimshaw NS, Murray EB. The acceptability of milk and milk products in populations with a high prevalence of lactose intolerance. *Am J Clin Nutr.* 1988;48(suppl):1086-1098.
10. Tong MJ, Strickland T, Votteri BA, Gunning JJ. Supplementary folates in the therapy of plasmodium falciparum malaria. *JAMA.* 1970;214:2330-2333.
11. *Facts and Comparisons.* 1988:1531-1533.
12. *USPDI.* 11th ed. 1991:2365-2368.
13. *Facts and Comparisons.* 1988:1523-1525.
14. Ogunbona FA, Smith IF, Olawoye OS. Fat contents of meals and bioavailability of griseofulvin in man. *J Pharm Pharmacol.* 1985;37:283-284.
15. Roe DA. *Alcohol and the Diet.* Westport, Conn: AVI Publ Co; 1979:217.
16. Lesher JL, Graham Smith J. Antifungal agents in dermatology. *J Am Acad Dermatol.* 1987;17:383-394.
17. *Facts and Comparisons.* 1988:1503-1504.
18. Mannisto PT, Mantyla R, Nykanen S, et al. Impairing effect of food on ketoconazole absorption. *Antimicrob Agents Chemother.* 1982;21:730.
19. Kraemer FB, Pont A. Inhibition of cholesterol synthesis by ketoconazole. *Am J Med.* 1986;80:616-622.
20. Graybill JR, Craven PC. Antifungal agents used in systemic mycoses: activity and therapeutic use. *Drugs.* 1983;25:41-62.
21. *USPDI.* 11th ed. 1991:172-175.
22. *Facts and Comparisons.* 1988:1505-1507.

Section X
Genitourinary Disease and Contraception

SECTION

X GENITOURINARY DISEASE AND CONTRACEPTION

X.1. URINARY INFECTIONS

A. *Drugs used in primary disease control*

GENERIC NAME	BRAND NAME	ASSOCIATED DNI	REFERENCE
Methenamine (Antibacterial)	**Mandelamine** (Parke-Davis)	Product may contain tartrazine, which can induce hives or asthma in patients sensitive to foods containing tartrazine.	1
		An acid pH of the urine should be maintained during treatment; may be attained by giving cranberry juice.	2
		The oral suspension is incompatible with enteral formulas.	3
Nitrofurantoin (Antibacterial)	**Furadantin** (Norwich Eaton)	Should be given with milk or food to avoid gastric upset.	4

GENERIC NAME	BRAND NAME	ASSOCIATED DNI	REFERENCE
		Better absorbed when taken with food.	5
		Contains sorbitol, which may cause diarrhea.	
Tetracycline (Antibiotic)	**Achromycin V** (Lederle) **Panmycin** (Upjohn) **Robitet** (Robins) **Sumycin** (Squibb)	See Section II.2.A.	

Risk factors related to lack of primary disease control in patients with urinary infections

Risk of lack of disease control in patients on Mandelamine may be related to diets that are not associated with production of an acid urine.

X.2.
CONTRACEPTION

GENERIC NAME	BRAND NAME	ASSOCIATED DNI	REFERENCE
Ethinyl estradiol + norgestrel (Oral contraceptive)	**Ovral** (Wyeth)	Folate and vitamin B_6 requirements may be increased by this and other oral contraceptives.	6

GENERIC NAME	BRAND NAME	ASSOCIATED DNI	REFERENCE
		Riboflavin depletion has been reported in malnourished women on oral contraceptives, but does not develop in US women on RDA or >RDA intakes of the vitamin.	7

Risk factors for vitamin depletion in patients using oral contraceptives

Risk factors include mineral intake of folate or vitamin B_6, malabsorption states including gluten-sensitive enteropathy, and inflammatory bowel disease.

SECTION X REFERENCES

1. *Facts and Comparisons.* 1988:1616.
2. Hansten PD. *Drug Interactions.* 5th ed. Philadelphia: Lea & Febiger; 1985: 219-220.
3. Roe DA. *Diet and Drug Interactions.* New York: Van Nostrand Reinhold; 1988:38.
4. *Facts and Comparisons.* 1988:1612-1614.
5. Rosenberg HA, Bates TR. The influence of food on nitrofurantoin bioavailability. *Clin Pharmacol Ther.* 1976;20:227-229.
6. Roe DA. Nutrition and the contraceptive pill. In: Winick M, ed. *Nutritional Disorders of American Women.* New York: John Wiley & Sons; 1977:37-49.
7. Oral contraceptives and nutrient interactions. *Indian Council Med Res Bull.* 1985;15:85-89.

Appendixes

Appendix

A

Intervention Index

Additional drug-nutrient interactions related to drugs are listed in the earlier sections of this manual.

DRUG	DNI	WHAT TO DO	TESTS
Acetohexamide	Diuresis and dehydration	Stop drug if patient is dehydrated.	Hematocrit
Albuterol	Hyperglycemia	Stop drug if patient is diabetic.	Blood glucose
Allopurinol	Drug rash	Stop drug.	Drug level
	Blood loss at surgery	Stop warfarin therapy.	Prothrombin time
Aluminum hydroxide	Low absorption of tetracycline	Stop drug.	Tetracycline level
	Osteomalacia	Stop drug; prescribe vitamin D supplement.	X-ray; serum phosphate
Amantadine	Dry mouth and constipation	Increase fluids and fiber.	None
Amiloride	Hyperkalemia; hyponatremia; anorexia	Stop drug.*	Serum potassium; chemical profile
Amiodarone	Weight gain and hypothyroidism	Stop drug.*	Weight; T_3; T_4
Amoxicillin	Slow therapy effect	Give with increased fluids.	Temperature
Amphotericin B	Renal failure	Stop drug; use dialysis.	Serum potassium; magnesium and blood urea nitrogen

DRUG	DNI	WHAT TO DO	TESTS
Aspirin	Low hemoglobin	Stop drug; check GI blood loss.	CBC; serum iron
	Low plasma folate	Stop drug.	Plasma and RBC folate
Atenolol		See propranolol.	
Azidothymidine	Anorexia; megaloblastic anemia	Stop drug.	WBC; RBC; serum folate
Azithromycin	Nausea, vomiting	Should be taken 1 hr before meal.	None
Benztropine	See Amantadine.		
Bisacodyl	See Phenolphthalein.		
Bleomycin	Low food intake	Give oral formula.	Monitor weight
Bromocriptine	Anorexia; nausea	Reduce dose of Sinemet.	None
Bumetanide		See Furosemide.	
Calcium carbonate	Milk-alkali syndrome	Stop calcium carbonate.	Serum calcium; x-ray
	Low iron absorption	Stop calcium supplements.	CBC; serum ferritin
Captopril	No taste; anorexia; weight loss	Change to enalapril.	Monitor weight.
Carbamazepine	Anorexia and stomatitis	Stop drug; give transfusion.	CBC
	Taste distortion	Stop drug if weight loss occurs.	Body weight
Carbidopa and levodopa	Less risk of vitamin B_6 deficiency	Use Sinemet instead of carbidopa and levodopa.	
Carmustine	Hepatic injury Nephropathy	Stop drug.	Serum alkaline phosphatase and blood urea nitrogen
Chloroquine	Hemolytic anemia	Check if G6PD deficient.	RBC; G6PD

DRUG	DNI	WHAT TO DO	TESTS
Chlorpromazine	Hyperphagia and weight gain	Reduce food access.	Monitor weight.
	Edema and hyponatremia	Reduce dose; increase salt intake.	Weight; serum sodium
	Riboflavin depletion	Increase milk; prescribe B_2 supplements.	Erythrocyte glutathione reductase assay
Chlorpropamide	Weight gain	Stop drug if weight gain due to edema.	Serum sodium
	Hypoglycemia	Use short-acting oral drug.	Blood glucose
	Flush	Advise abstention from alcohol.	None
Cholestyramine	Folate deficiency; vitamin A, D, and K deficiency	Lower dose; give vitamin supplements.	Prothrombin time; serum and RBC folate; assess status for vitamins A, D, and K
Cimetidine	Bleeding with warfarin	Stop cimetidine; give vitamin K.	Prothrombin time
	Lack of drug effect	Stop antacids.	None
	Alcoholic intoxication	Advise abstention from alcohol.	None
	Vitamin B_{12} depletion	Give vitamin B_{12} orally or im.	Serum vitamin B_{12}; CBC
Cisplatin	Nephrotoxicity; magnesium deficiency	Provide pretherapy iv hydration.	Serum magnesium; calcium; blood urea nitrogen
Clofibrate	Nausea; vitamin K deficiency	Stop drugs.	Prothrombin time; hemoglobin
Clonidine	Hyperglycemia: dry mouth	Stop drug in diabetics.	Blood glucose

DRUG	DNI	WHAT TO DO	TESTS
Colchicine	Weight loss	Stop drug; possible malabsorption.	Serum folate and B_{12}
Colestipol		See Cholestyramine.	
Cromolyn sodium	Nausea	Stop drug.	None
Cyclophos-phamide	Vomiting and diarrhea	Give small, frequent feedings.	Monitor weight.
Cyclosporine	Gouty attack if history Renal impairment	Give low-purine diet; advise salt restriction and liberal fluid intake.	BP Serum uric acid Lipid levels
	Elevated triglycerides	Advise adequate caloric intake with moderation in fat and simple sugars.	
Dactinomycin	Nausea and stomatitis	Give formula foods.	Monitor weight.
Diazepam	Dry mouth	Reduce dose.	None
Digoxin	Anorexia and weight loss	Reduce dose or stop drug.	ECG; serum potassium: weight
Diltiazem		See Nifedipine.	
Diphenoxylate with atropine	Dry mouth	Give ice to suck.	None
Disulfiram	Disulfiram reaction	Advise abstention from alcohol.	None
Doxorubicin	Cardiomyopathy	Stop drug; prescribe vitamin E and B_2.	Pulse: ECG
Enalapril	Dry mouth; GI symptoms	Lower dose.	Monitor weight.
Encainide	Hyperglycemia: anorexia	Stop drug.	Blood glucose
Erythromycin	Slow therapeutic effect	If stearate, give fasting.	None

DRUG	DNI	WHAT TO DO	TESTS
Ethacrynic acid		See Furosemide.	
Ethambutol	Gouty attack if history	Stop drug; treat gout.	Serum uric acid
	Nausea	Give with food.	None
	Visual impairment	Stop drug.	Blood glucose
Etretinate	Anorexia and dysgeusia	Stop drug.	Monitor weight.
	See Isotretinoin.		
	Increased absorption with milk	Give with milk if patient can tolerate.	Drug level
Famotidine	No bleeding with warfarin		
Felodipine	Flush	Avoid taking with grapefruit juice. Take with a low-fat meal.	
5-Fluorouracil	Anorexia and stomatitis	Give formula foods.	Monitor weight.
Fluphenazine	See Chlorpromazine.		
Flurazepam	See Lorazepam.		
Furosemide	Electrolyte imbalance: digoxin toxicity	Stop drug; give potassium supplement.	Serum potassium; sodium: ECG
Gemfibrozil	Dry mouth; anorexia	Check weight change.	None
Gentamicin	Hypokalemia	Stop drug.	Serum potassium and magnesium; blood urea nitrogen
Glipizide	Less postprandial elevated glucose	Use drug in elderly patients with diabetes.	Blood glucose
Glyburide	Nocturnal hypoglycemia	Stop drug; start glipizide therapy; give late-night snack.	Morning blood glucose

DRUG	DNI	WHAT TO DO	TESTS
Gold sodium thiomalate	Hypoalbuminemia	Stop drug; check renal function.	Serum and urine albumin
Griseofulvin	Lack of effect	Give with small amount of corn oil.	Drug level
	Flush and headache	Tell patient to avoid alcohol.	None
Guanabenz	Dry mouth; bad taste	Promote fluid intake.	None
Guanethidine	Weight gain due to edema	Lower dose or stop drug.	Monitor weight.
Haloperidol	Constipation	Add bran to diet; push fluids.	None
Hydralazine	Vitamin B_6 deficiency; sensitivity to tartrazine	Give with B_6; give if no sensitivity to tartrazine.	B_6 assays
Hydrochlorothia-zide	Hyponatremia	Stop drug; increase sodium intake.	Serum sodium
	Hypokalemia	Lower dose and add potassium supplements.	Serum potassium
	Hyperglycemia	Stop drug in diabetics.	Blood glucose
	Hyperlipidemia	Stop drug.	Serum cholesterol; low-density lipoproteins
	Gout	Stop drug; treat gout.	Serum uric acid
Imipramine	Riboflavin depletion	Increase milk intake.	Erythrocyte glutathione reductase test on RBC
Insulin	Hypoglycemia	Give glucose orally or iv.	Blood glucose
Iodinated glycerol	Flush	Stop drug.	None
Isoetharine	Allergic reaction	Stop drug.	None

DRUG	DNI	WHAT TO DO	TESTS
Isoniazid	Lack of TB control	Give fasting.	Chest x-ray; examine sputum
	Neuropathy	Give with B_6 supplements (25 mg).	Plasma B_6 phosphate
	Seizures	Give vitamin B_6 iv.	Vital signs
	Pellagra	Give B_6, plus niacin.	Urine assays
	Osteomalacia; rickets	Give vitamin D supplements and UV exposure.	Serum 25-OH-cholecalciferol; serum calcium
Isotretinoin	Acute pancreatitis	Stop drug; treat emergency.	Serum amylase
	Nausea and jaundice	Stop drug; stop alcohol.	Serum glutamic-oxaloacetic transaminase; serum glutamic-pyruvic transaminase
	Food increases absorption.	Give with food.	Drug level
	Birth defects	Check risk of pregnancy before initiating therapy.	Check if pregnant.
	Hyperlipidemia	Reduce fat and cholesterol intake.	Serum triglycerides and cholesterol
	Back pain	Reduce dose or stop drug.	X-ray spine

DRUG	DNI	WHAT TO DO	TESTS
Ketoconazole	Nausea	Stop drug.	Serum glutamic-oxaloacetic transaminase; serum glutamic-pyruvic transaminase
	Liver damage in infants	Do not give if lactating.	Drug in milk
Labetalol		See Propranolol.	
Lactulose	Reduced blood ammonia	Continue drug.	Blood ammonia
	Loss of water-soluble vitamins, electrolytes	MVI to meet RDAs.	Monitor electrolytes.
Levodopa	Anorexia	Give with carbidopa.	Body weight
	Nausea	Give with food but not with meat.	None
	Hypokalemia	Give potassium supplement.	Serum potassium
	Neuritis due to B_6 deficiency	Reduce dose; give vitamin B_6 supplement.	Plasma B_6 phosphate
	Tyramine reaction	Advise patient to abstain from cheese during therapy with monoamine oxidase inhibitors.	Blood pressure
	Hives and asthma	Stop drug; change brand.	None
	Loss of drug effect	Stop vitamin B_6 supplement.	Rigidity test
Lithium carbonate	Loss of mania control	Reduce salt intake.	Blood lithium

DRUG	DNI	WHAT TO DO	TESTS
	Weight gain without edema	Remove snacks; reduce calories.	Body weight
	Nausea; weight gain; edema	Stop drug; give more sodium.	Lithium level
Lomustine	Nausea and vomiting	Stop food for 3 hours after therapy.	None
Loperamide	Electrolyte imbalance	Stop drug.	Serum electrolytes
Lorazepam	Low food intake; sleepiness	Reduce dose.	Monitor weight.
Lovastatin	GI symptoms: absorption best with food	Give with food.	None
Magnesium hydroxide	Hypotension; respiratory failure	Stop drug; use dialysis in patient who is hypotensive.	Serum magnesium; blood urea nitrogen
Magnesium sulfate	Dehydration and hypermagnese-mia	Stop drug; give iv fluids.	Serum magnesium
Methenamine	Blocked nasogastric tube	Do not give via ng tube.	Check flow in ng tube.
	Lack of drug effect	Give with cranberry juice.	pH of urine
	Hives or asthma	Stop drug.	None
Methotrexate	Weight loss with folate deficiency	Give folinic acid if drug nutrient interaction is acute.	CBC; serum and RBC folate
Methoxsalen	Nausea and dyspepsia	Give with milk.	None
Methyldopa	Drug absorption slow with iron or protein	Give with low-protein food & not with iron supplement.	Monitor blood pressure.
Methylphenidate	Growth retardation	Stop drug; increase caloric intake.	Weight and height

DRUG	DNI	WHAT TO DO	TESTS
Metoclopramide	Altered drug and nutrient absorption	Check blood glucose and drug levels.	Blood glucose; serum drug level
Metoprolol		See Propranolol.	
Metronidazole	Disulfiram reaction	Tell patient no alcohol.	None
Mineral oil	Fat-soluble vitamin deficiency	Stop drug; give supplemental vitamins A, D, and K.	Prothrombin time; 25-OH-cholecalciferol
Minoxidil	Weight gain due to edema	Lower dose or stop drug.	Monitor weight.
Misoprostol	Nausea; dyspepsia; diarrhea	Give after meals and at bedtime.	None
Morphine	Anorexia; constipation	Give high-fiber diet.	None
Moxalactam	Vitamin K deficiency with bleeding	Stop drug; give vitamin K im.	Prothrombin time
Nadolol		See Propranolol.	
Naproxen and other NSAIDs	Hyperkalemia	Stop drug; check renal function.	Serum potassium; blood urea nitrogen
	Anemia	Stop drug; give iron therapy.	Blood in stool
	Weight gain with edema	Stop drug; check renal function.	Weight; blood urea nitrogen
Niacin	Flushing	Give amide or with aspirin.	None
Nifedipine	Flushing	Give drug with low-fat meal.	None
Nitrofurantoin	GI symptoms	Give with milk.	None
Nitroglycerin	Faintness with alcohol	Warn against drinking alcohol.	Blood pressure
Olsalazine	Diarrhea	Take with food.	WBC
Omeprazole	Dry mouth	Increase fluids. Do not chew capsule.	None

DRUG	DNI	WHAT TO DO	TESTS
Oral contraceptives	Folate and vitamin B_6 depleted	Advise high-folate and B_6 diet.	Serum and RBC folate; serum B_6
Oxytetracycline	Slow therapeutic effect	Avoid milk and dairy products, Ca and Fe supplements, antacids, and Mg-containing laxatives 1 hr before and after dose.	None
Pancrelipase	Reduced steatorrhea	Give before meal.	Fecal fat
	Folate depletion	Give folate supplements.	Serum and RBC folate
Paramethadione	Hives or asthma	Stop drug.	None
Penicillamine	Loss of taste	Stop drug; check if low in zinc.	Serum and RBC zinc
	Neuritis with vitamin B_6 deficiency	Stop drug; give vitamin B_6 supplements.	Plasma B_6
Pentamidine	Hyperglycemia or hypoglycemia	Give with iv glucose if patient is hypoglycemic.	Blood glucose
	Megaloblastic anemia	Give drug with folate supplement.	CBC; serum and RBC folate
Pentoxifylline	Anorexia; dry mouth	Check food intake and weight change.	Monitor weight.
	Anorexia and nausea	Reduce dose or stop drug.	Check body weight.
Perphenazine	See Chlorpromazine.		
Phenelzine	Tyramine reaction	Avoid aged cheese.	Monitor blood pressure.
Phenobarbital	Coma	Start hemodialysis.	Drug and alcohol level
Phenolphthalein	Weight loss	Check for steatorrhea.	Fecal fat; weight

DRUG	DNI	WHAT TO DO	TESTS
	Hypokalemia	Stop drug; give iv potassium.	Serum potassium
Phenytoin	Bleeding at surgery	Stop warfarin; administer vitamin K.	Prothrombin time
	Loss of seizure control	Stop folate.	Drug level
	Neonatal hemorrhage	Give vitamin K.	Prothrombin time
	Rickets/ osteomalacia	Give vitamin D supplements.	Serum calcium; serum 25-OH-cholecalciferol
	Incompatible with formula	Give drug without formula infusion.	Drug level
	Macrocytic anemia	Give less than 5 mg folic acid/ day.	CBC; serum and RBC folate
	Slow to control seizures	Increase dose if obese.	Drug level
Pindolol	Does not affect triglycerides.	See Propranolol.	
Potassium iodide with niacin	Flush	Stop drug.	None
	Hyperkalemia	Stop drug.	Serum potassium; blood urea nitrogen
Prazosin	Weight gain due to edema	Lower dose.	Monitor weight.
Prednisone	Poor growth	Reduce dose.	Weight for height
	Osteoporosis	Reduce dose; give calcium supplement.	X-rays of bone density
	Weight gain	Lower dose; decrease caloric and salt intake.	Monitor weight.
	Hyperglycemia	Lower dose if diabetic.	Blood glucose; glycosylated hemoglobin

DRUG	DNI	WHAT TO DO	TESTS
Primidone	Megaloblastic anemia	Give folate supplements.	RBC; mean corpuscular volume; serum folate
Probenecid	Renal colic with stones	Stop drug; give fluids.	X-ray; urine pH
Probucol	Anorexia; slow absorption	Give after food.	Weight; serum lipids
Procainamide	Anorexia and nausea	Stop drug or lower dose.	ECG; blood urea nitrogen
Procarbazine	Vitamin B_6 deficiency	Give with 25 mg/day B_6.	Plasma B_6 phosphate
	Tyramine reaction	Advise patient to abstain from cheese during therapy with monoamine oxidase inhibitors.	Blood pressure
Prochlorperazine	Good effect, less nausea	Give rectally if patient becomes nauseated.	None
Propantheline bromide	Promotes absorption of vitamin B_2 and drug.	Check drug levels in serum.	Serum drug levels
	Dry mouth	Reduce dose.	None
Propranolol	Hypoglycemia in diabetics	Stop drug; give glucose.	Blood glucose
	Increases triglycerides.	Change to Pindolol.	Serum lipids
	Low blood level of drug	Give with food.	Drug level
	CNS side effects	Reduce dose; treat malnutrition.	Serum albumin
Psyllium gum	Anorexia and bloating	Stop drug.	Monitor weight.
	Riboflavin depletion	Stop drug.	Erythrocyte glutathione reductase

DRUG	DNI	WHAT TO DO	TESTS
Pyrazinamide	Pellagra with niacin deficiency	Give niacin and vitamin B_6 supplements.	Urine assays
	Neuritis with B_6 deficiency	Give vitamin B_6 supplements with drug.	Plasma B_6 phosphate
Pyrimethamine	Megaloblastic anemia	Stop drug; give folate supplement.	CBC; serum and RBC folate
Quinidine	Vitamin K deficiency with anticoagulants	Stop drug; give vitamin K.	Prothrombin time; hemoglobin
Ranitidine	Vitamin B_{12} depletion	Give vitamin V_{12} orally or im.	CBC; serum B_{12}
	Bleeding with warfarin	Stop drug; give vitamin K.	Prothrombin time
Rauwolfia	Anorexia; weight gain with edema	Stop drug.	Monitor weight.
Rifampin	Loss of drug effect	Give drug fasting.	None
	Vitamin B_{12} and folate test problem	Use alternate assays.	Serum B_2 and serum folate
	Vitamin D deficiency	Give vitamin D supplement if patient cannot tolerate milk.	Serum 25-OH-cholecalciferol; serum calcium
Senna	See Phenolphthalein.		
Sodium bicarbonate	Milk-alkali syndrome	Stop drug; lower calcium intake.	Serum calcium; blood urea nitrogen
	Folate deficiency	Stop drug; give folate supplement.	Serum and RBC folate; CBC
	Heart failure with edema	Stop drug; administer diuretic.	Serum sodium; weight; ECG

DRUG	DNI	WHAT TO DO	TESTS
Sodium chloride	Used for salt depletion	Take salt if exercising.	Serum sodium and chloride
Spironolactone	Hyperkalemia; hypernatremia	Stop drug.	Serum potassium; sodium; blood urea nitrogen
	Hypo-phosphatemia	Replace phosphate as indicated.	Monitor serum phosphate levels.
Sucralfate	Low absorption of digoxin and phenytoin	Give 2 hours after digoxin or phenytoin; do not give with aluminum hydroxide due to risk of hypophosphatemia.	Drug levels
Sulfadoxine/ pyrimethidine	Megaloblastic anemia	Give folinic acid CBC and or folic acid serum plus.	RBC folate
	Stomatitis	Give with formula foods.	Monitor weight.
	Hypoglycemia in diabetic patients	Stop drug; give iv glucose.	Blood glucose
Sulfasalazine	Folate deficiency	Stop drug; give folic acid.	CBC; serum and RBC folate
Sulindac	Urticaria (hives)	Stop drug.	None
Tamoxifen	Hypercalcemia	Do not give if blood urea nitrogen level is high.	Serum calcium; blood urea nitrogen
Temazepam	See Lorazepam.		

DRUG	DNI	WHAT TO DO	TESTS
Tetracycline	Slow therapeutic effect	Avoid milk and dairy products, Ca and Fe supplements, antacids, and Mg-containing laxatives 1 hr before and after dose.	None
Theophylline	Dizziness	Avoid giving drug with high-fat meal.	Drug level
	Wheezing	Stop high-protein supplement or diet.	Drug level
	Anorexia and weight loss	Lower dose.	Drug level; weight
	Insomnia; arrhythmia	Stop caffeine beverages.	ECG
Thioridazine	Blocked nasogastric tube	Replace nasogastric tube.	Drug level
	See Chlorpromazine.		
Thiothixene	See Chlorpromazine.		
Timolol	See Propranolol.		
Tolazamide	Hypoglycemia	Stop drug; administer glipizide.	Blood glucose
Tolbutamide	False-positive reaction for albumin in urine	Stop drug; recheck urine.	Renal function
Triamterene	Hyperkalemia; folate deficiency	Stop drug; give folic acid.	Serum potassium; serum plus RBC folate
Trimethoprim	Folate deficiency; anemia	Stop drug; give folic acid.	Serum plus RBC folate

DRUG	DNI	WHAT TO DO	TESTS
Trimetrexate	Anemia; pancytopenia	Give folinic acid.	CBC; serum plus RBC folate
Valproic acid	Comatose condition	Stop drug; give carnitine.	Liver panel
	Bleeding	Stop drug if surgery planned.	Bleeding time
	Drug in breast milk	Stop if breast feeding.	Drug in milk
Verapamil	Lowered drug effect with calcium	Stop calcium supplement.	ECG; pulse
Vincristine	Nausea and constipation	Give formula with fiber.	Monitor weight.
Vitamin A	Retinol toxicity	Stop vitamin A supplement.	Serum retinol
Warfarin	Vitamin K deficiency with bleeding	Stop drug; give vitamin K injections.	Prothrombin time; hemoglobin

*When drug is stopped, an alternative with similar therapeutic effect or an alternate dose form should be considered.

Appendix B
Algorithms

Drug and Nutrient Problem Diagnosis and Solution in Cardiac and Hypertensive Patients

Problem 1: Acute Confusion

Drug causes are (a) digitalis toxicity and (b) hyponatremia.

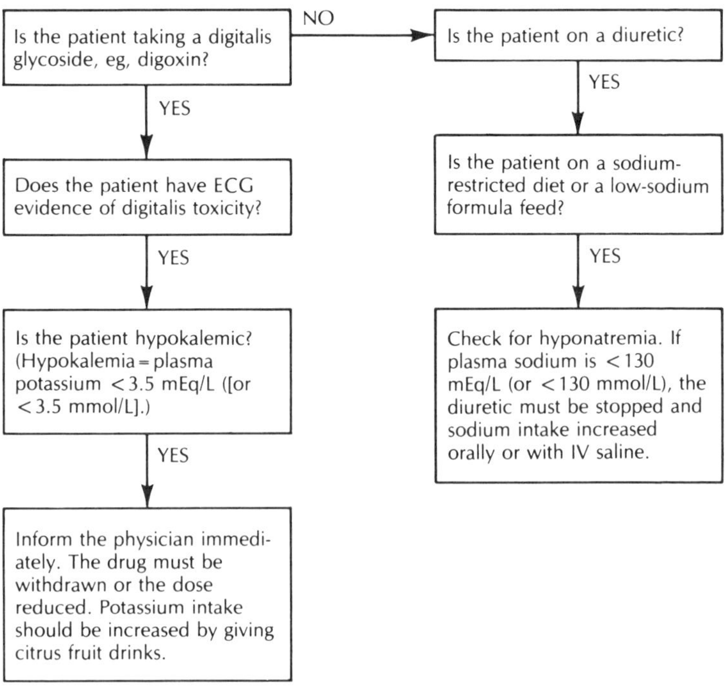

Problem 2: Weight Loss

Weight loss in a patient with cardiac disease can be due to loss of edema or of fat and muscle.

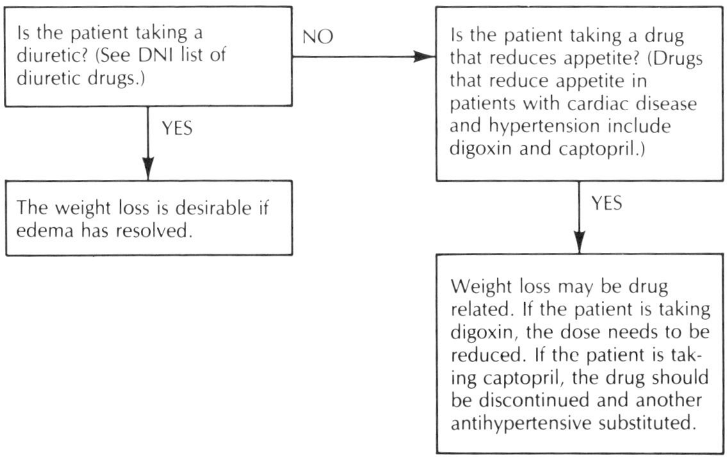

Problem 3: Weight Gain

Weight gain is due to edema or gain in fat and lean body mass.

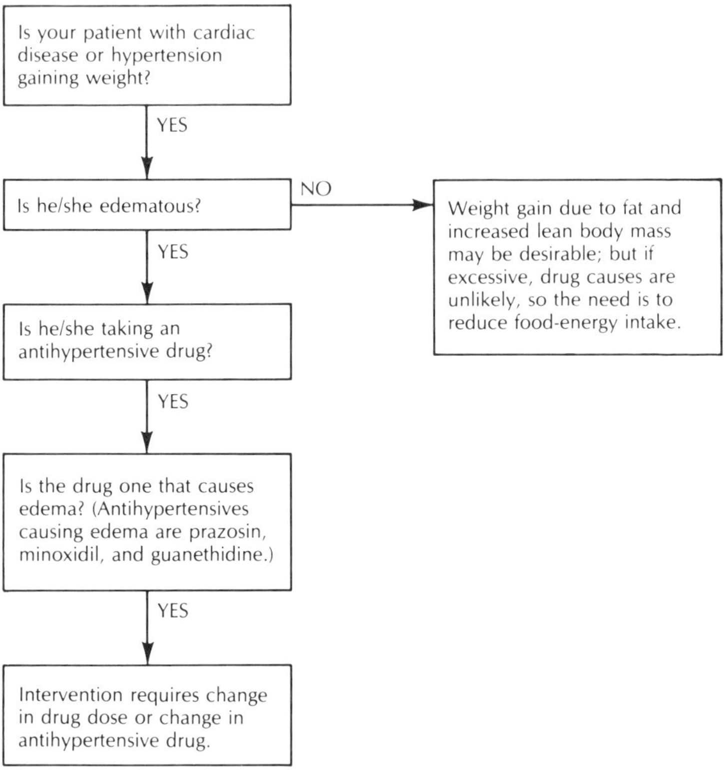

Drug and Nutrient Interactions in Diabetic Patients

Problem 1: Acute Confusion

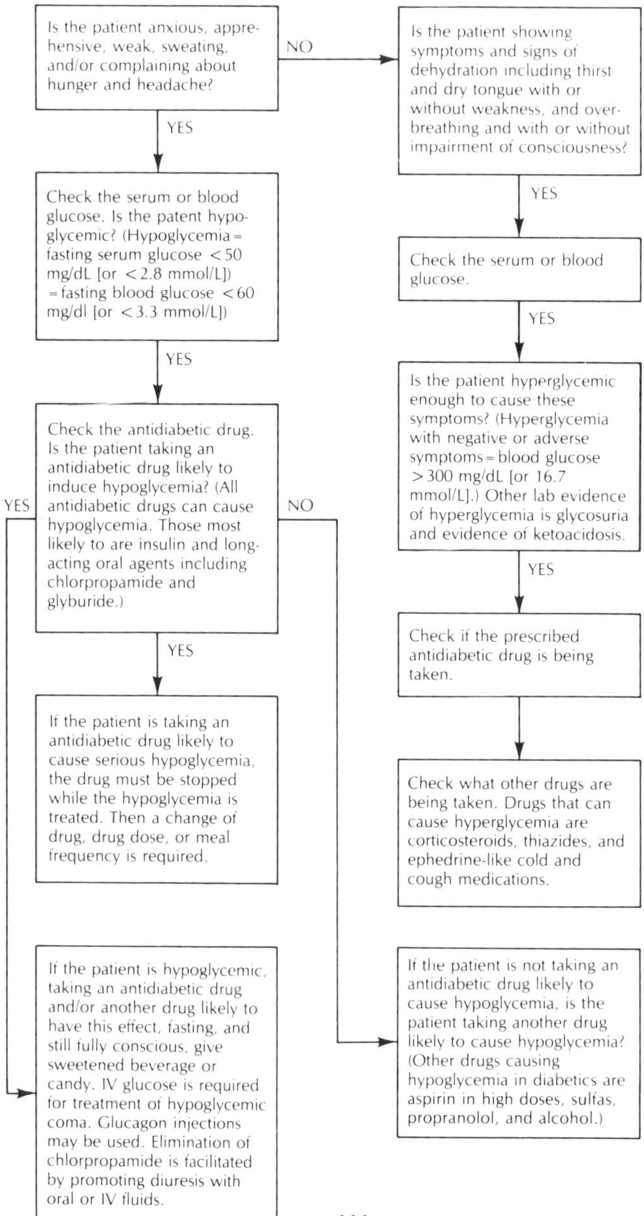

Problem 2: Flush

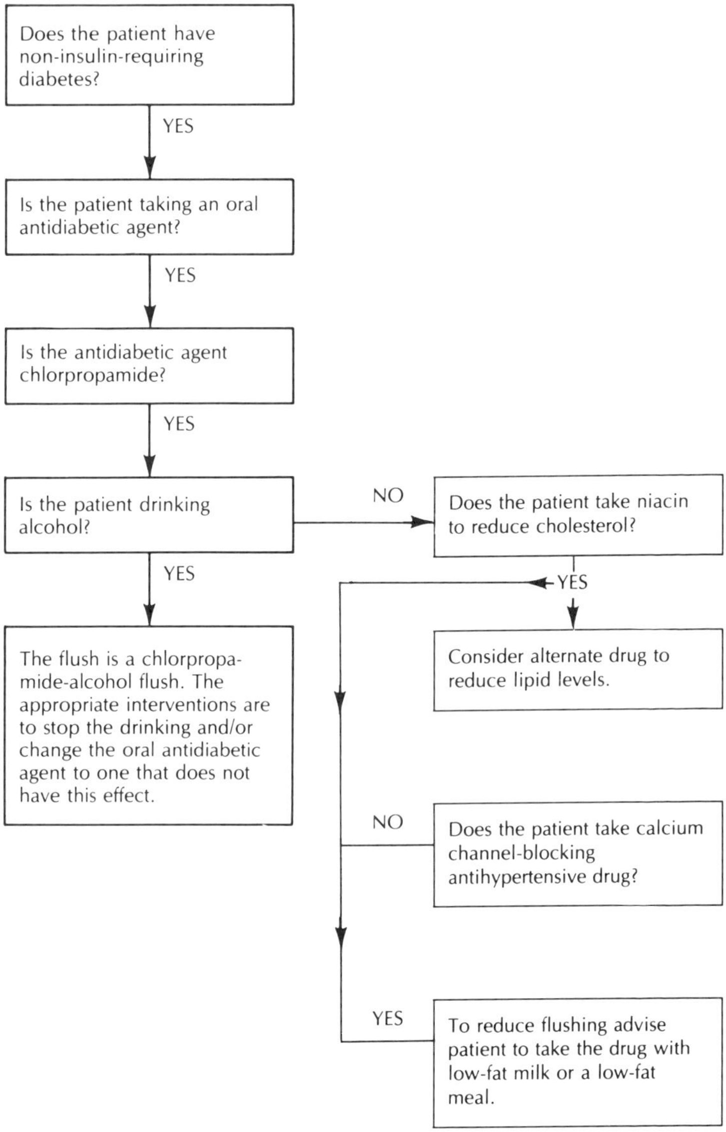

Drugs and Weight Gain

Weight gain can result from additional fat, fluid, or lean body mass.

Consider the drugs associated with weight gain as fat, as edema fluid and as lean body mass ("muscle").

Fat
Chlorpromazine and other phenothiazines
Prednisone and other corticosteroids

Fluid
Minoxidil
Guanadrel
Guanethidine
Methyldopa
Lithium
Chlorpromazine
Chlorpropamide
Corticosteroids

Muscle
Insulin
Antibiotics
Anticancer drugs

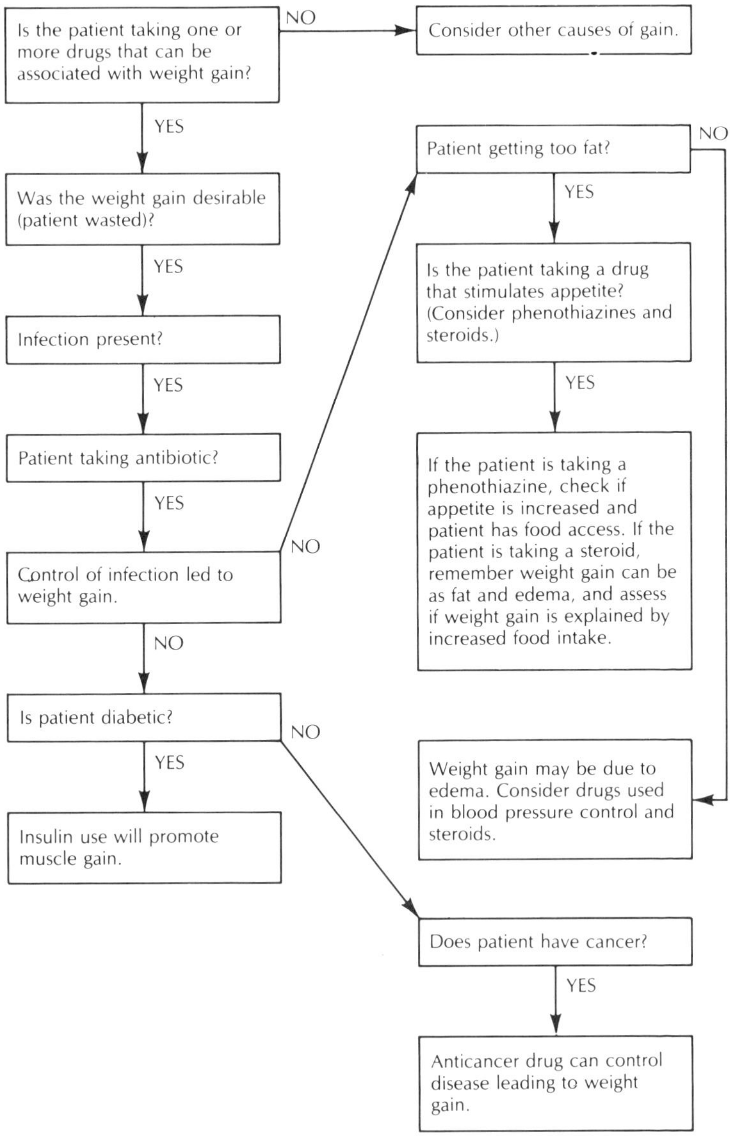
Is the patient taking one or more drugs that can be associated with weight gain?
NO
Consider other causes of gain.
YES
Was the weight gain desirable (patient wasted)?
YES
Infection present?
YES
Patient taking antibiotic?
YES
Control of infection led to weight gain.
NO
Patient getting too fat?
YES
Is the patient taking a drug that stimulates appetite? (Consider phenothiazines and steroids.)
YES
If the patient is taking a phenothiazine, check if appetite is increased and patient has food access. If the patient is taking a steroid, remember weight gain can be as fat and edema, and assess if weight gain is explained by increased food intake.
NO
Weight gain may be due to edema. Consider drugs used in blood pressure control and steroids.
NO
Is patient diabetic?
YES
Insulin use will promote muscle gain.
NO
Does patient have cancer?
YES
Anticancer drug can control disease leading to weight gain.

Drugs and Weight Loss

Did the patient lose fat, fluid, or lean body mass?

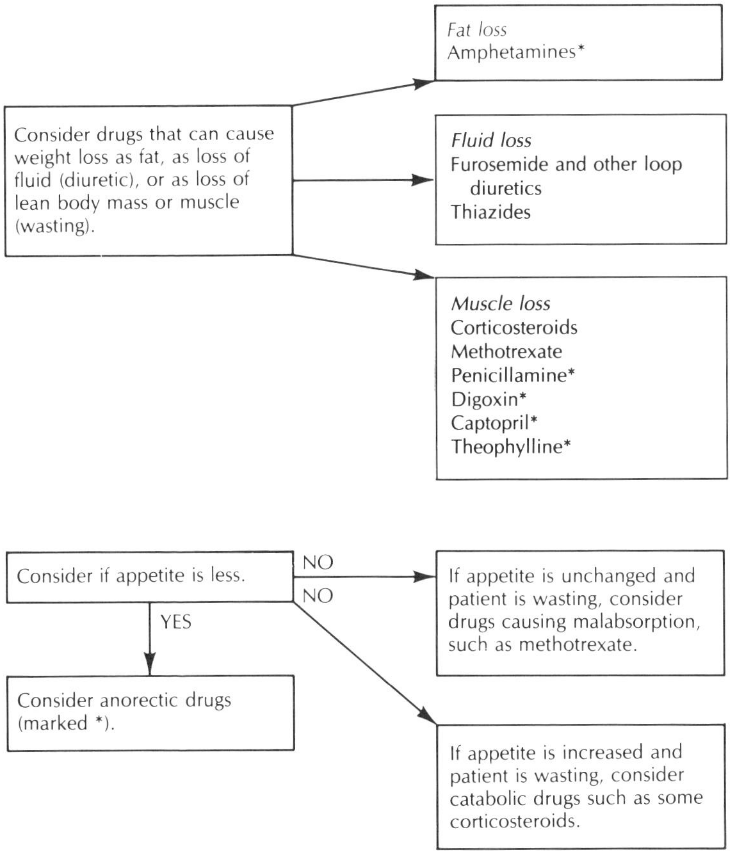

Drugs and Anemia

Consider drugs causing GI blood loss (low hemoglobin and low mean corpuscular volume [MCV]), as well as those causing megaloblastic anemia (low hemoglobin, low RBC, and high MCV).

With GI blood loss (low MCV/ iron deficiency anemia)
Aspirin
Indomethacin
Other NSAIDs
Valproic acid

Without GI blood loss (high MCV/folate deficiency anemia)
Methotrexate
Trimetrexate
Pyrimethamine
Trimethoprim
Triamterene
Phenytoin

With GI loss (increased MCV/ B_{12} deficiency)
Cimetidine
Ranitidine
Fanotidine

Exclude non-drug causes of blood loss.

Those related to diet (low iron intake and low folate intake).

Those related to disease (blood loss due to GI cancer, peptic ulcer, or megaloblastic anemia due to malabsorption, hemolysis, or bone marrow suppression).

Loss of Disease Control and Diet Risk

Loss of disease control is defined as a new state of disease activity in a disease previously made inactive or recurrence or spread of the disease.

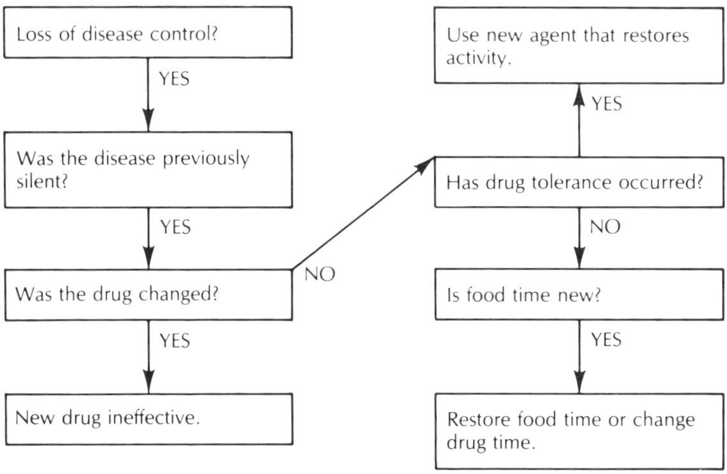

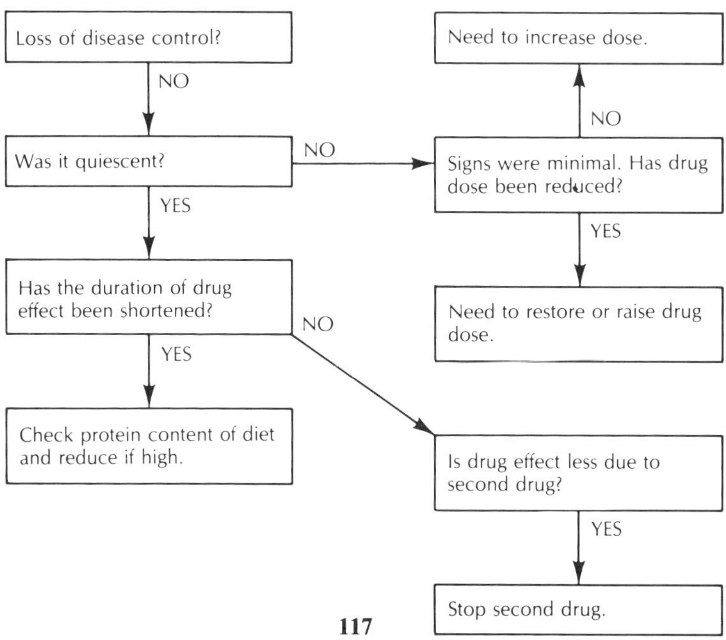

disease silent =disease present without symptoms or signs.
disease quiescent =disease present without symptoms.
disease recurrent =disease active, with signs present, after period of inactivity.
disease spread =spread to other organs or tissues either by direct invasion or spread via blood or lymphatic system.

Examples of loss of disease control and means to overcome:

1. Nitrate tolerance in patients with cardiac disease. Tolerance can be restored by giving a source of cysteine such as acetylcysteine, which is converted to cysteine in the body so allowing activation of guanylate cyclase. This enzyme increases the amount of cyclic guanosine monophosphate in smooth muscle, thus permitting vasodilator activity of drug.
2. Theophylline failure to control wheezing in patients with asthma. Activity of drug can be restored by reducing dietary protein content.
3. Phenytoin failure in seizure disorders. Failure can be due to high intake of folic acid, which should be stopped.
4. Sulfonylurea (oral antidiabetic agent) failure to achieve glycemic control in patients with diabetes. Failure can be due to thiazide, which is diabetogenic. Thiazide should be stopped and replaced with another antihypertensive agent that is not diabetogenic.

Appendix

C

Patient Instructions for Avoidance of Drug and Nutrient Interactions

A. *For cardiac patients*

1. *Information on digoxin and other preparations of digitalis*

   This medication (sometimes called a heart pill) has been prescribed to help your heart function more efficiently.

   a. Always take the medicine at the same time each day.
   b. Most patients should take their medicine one hour before breakfast.
   c. If you need to take your medicine with breakfast, eat similar breakfast foods every day.
   d. Do not include bran in the meal that accompanies or follows your medication.
   e. Do not stop taking the medicine unless you have checked this with your physician.
   f. Watch for signs of overdose. Important signs of overdose that you should report to your physician immediately are
      - Loss of appetite
      - Nausea and vomiting
      - Weight loss
      - Extreme tiredness
      - Slow, fast, or irregular pulse
      - Blurred or yellow vision
      - Drowsiness, depression, or confusion

2. *Information on diuretics: furosemide (Lasix), bumetanide (Bumex) and ethacrynic acid (Edecrin)*

   This medication (sometimes called a fluid pill) has been prescribed to help keep you from retaining fluid and the swelling of the legs and weight gain that can result. The following precautions are necessary if this medication is to be taken effectively and safely.

   a. Avoid eating high-sodium foods, including canned soup,

dried soup mixes, pickles, ketchup, green and ripe olives, relish, soy sauce, frankfurters, ham, bacon, corned beef, cold cuts, salted nuts, salted snack foods (such as potato chips), and Chinese food, unless it is prepared without salt and soy sauce.

b. Be sure to include vegetables and fruits (such as bananas and fruit juice) in your diet every day to ensure that you get food sources of potassium.

c. If you have been prescribed a potassium supplement, take it as directed, but do not use a potassium-containing salt substitute.

d. Take the medicine at the same time every day.

e. If the medicine upsets your stomach, take it with food.

f. To prevent loss of too much water or potassium in your body, tell your physician if you become sick, especially with vomiting or diarrhea.

   Signs of loss of too much potassium are

   - Weakness of your muscles
   - Mood changes
   - Confusion

g. To prevent loss of too much sodium, tell your physician if you become sick with vomiting or diarrhea. Signs of loss of too much sodium are

   - Weakness
   - Severe mental confusion
   - Faintness

h. If you are taking one of the diuretics listed above, do not take over-the-counter medicines unless you have checked with your physician. It is particularly important to avoid sodium-containing antacids.

i. If you are taking one of these diuretics, be sure to tell all doctors who prescribe medicine for you.

   NOTE: It may be dangerous to take these diuretics with lithium. The loss of sodium that occurs due to diuretics can cause lithium to be retained in the body. This can lead to dangerous side effects, including kidney failure.

j. If you are taking one of the diuretics listed above, drink a glass of low-fat milk every day. The calcium and vitamin D in the milk will help to reduce the risk of losing large amounts of calcium in your urine—and the risk of osteoporosis—due to the diuretic.

3. *Information on nitrates*

This medication has been prescribed to treat your angina. The information given below, unless stated otherwise, applies to all preparations of nitroglycerin.

a. Always carry regular, rapidly acting nitrate pills with you in a small container in your purse or pocket.
b. Let these fast-acting tablets dissolve under your tongue; do not swallow them.
c. Do not take the slow-acting nitrates, such as slow-acting isosorbide dinitrate (Isordil), at meal times. The food may delay the rate at which the medicine is absorbed.
d. Apply nitropatches to your skin exactly as you have been directed.
e. All patients who are taking nitroglycerin or using nitropatches should avoid alcohol because of the risk of faintness.
f. Avoid eating hot dogs and processed meats, including ham and cold cuts, that contain nitrate. Eating these foods can give you a headache or make you flush.

B. *For patients with high blood pressure*

1. *Information on thiazides: hydrochlorothiazide (including Esidrix or HydroDIURIL) and others (eg, methyclothiazide or Enduron)*

The medication you have been prescribed is being given to control your blood pressure. It will also prevent fluid retention.

a. Take this medication at the same time every day.
b. It is best to take it after a meal such as breakfast, which has a relatively constant food composition.
c. Do not eat salty foods or add salt to your food.
d. Do not go on a very low calorie diet.
e. Be sure to eat fruit and drink fruit juices every day. You should also eat vegetables that are good sources of potassium, since thiazide medications remove potassium from your body.
f. This medication can increase blood sugar and may interfere with control of diabetes. If you have diabetes, you should not take this medication unless the physician who is responsible for your diabetes management approves.

g. If you are predisposed to gout, you should avoid this medication, since it can cause attacks of gout.
h. This medication can increase blood cholesterol levels. If you have high blood cholesterol and/or heart disease, you should not take this medicine.

2. *Information on other blood pressure medicine*

This medication is being given to you to reduce your blood pressure.

a. Certain blood pressure pills—including propranolol (Inderal) and hydralazine (Apresoline)—are best taken after you eat.
b. Certain blood pressure pills—including captopril (Capoten)—can reduce your sense of taste and can also severely reduce your appetite. The risk of your losing your appetite because of this medicine is greater if you are a senior and are also taking digoxin for your heart or theophylline for asthma.
c. Certain blood pressure pills—such as minoxidil (Loniten)—can cause you to gain weight. You should report this weight gain to your physician because it is due to fluid retention.
d. Certain blood pressure pills—such as hydralazine (Apresoline)—can cause weakness in your hands, due to a medication-induced deficiency of vitamin B_6. If you are taking this medicine, ask your physician if you should be taking a vitamin B_6 supplement as well. Do not, however, take a supplement with more vitamin B_6 than is in a daily multivitamin pill unless your physician recommends it.
e. Certain blood pressure medicine—including spironolactone (Aldactone), triamterene (Dyrenium), and amiloride (Midamor)—prevent potassium loss from your body. If you had been taking a thiazide and have switched to one or more of the blood pressure medications just cited, you should stop taking a potassium supplement. You should not use a salt substitute, and you should not take pain or arthritis pills like ibuprofen (Motrin) unless your physician prescribes them. These substances may make potassium build up in your body and interfere with your kidney function. Certain blood pressure pills called calcium channel blockers can make you flush. The risk of flushing is reduced by taking the medi-

cation with a low-fat meal and avoiding taking it with grapefruit.

C. *For patients with lung problems*

1. *Information on theophylline and other asthma medicine*

This medicine has been prescribed to control your wheezing and to let you breathe better.

a. When you are taking this medicine, do not make any major dietary changes unless your physician advises you to do so. The reason for sticking to your usual diet is that the dosage of theophylline you need to control your asthma has been based on that diet. If you eat more protein food than usual, the theophylline will control your wheezing for a shorter time. If you take the medicine with a high-fat meal, the theophylline may be absorbed too quickly and cause side effects.

b. If you have ever had a reaction to sulfites used in or on foods, tell your physician so that he or she will not prescribe an asthma aerosol nebulizer that contains sulfite, such as isoetharine.

2. *Information on medicine used in the treatment of bronchitis*

This medicine has been prescribed to treat your bronchitis.

a. If you have been prescribed amoxicillin, be sure to take it with plenty (more than 4 fluid oz) of water.

b. If you are taking Bactrim or Septra, be sure to include good sources of folic acid in your diet because this medicine increases your requirements for this vitamin. Good food sources of folic acid are dark green vegetables, such as spinach or broccoli.

3. *Information on medicines used in the treatment of tuberculosis*

This medicine (isoniazid) has been prescribed to control your tuberculosis. You should continue to take it until your physician tells you to stop.

a. While you are taking isoniazid, you also should take the vitamin B_6 supplement, which will prevent side effects.

b. While you are taking isoniazid, be sure to include meat and/or other protein foods in your daily diet, but avoid canned fish, such as tuna, which can give you a reaction.

D. *For patients with stomach or intestinal problems*

1. *Information on medicine used to treat peptic ulcer*

a. If you have been prescribed cimetidine (Tagamet), do not drink alcoholic beverages because you are at risk of getting intoxicated even with a very small drink.
b. If you take antacids, limit your intake to that advised by your doctor. A high intake of aluminum-containing, over-the-counter antacids can cause muscle weakness and bone disorders.

2. *Information on medicine used to treat cystic fibrosis*
   a. If you—or your child—have been prescribed a medicine such as pancreatin to aid digestion, be sure to take it before each meal.
   b. Take the vitamin supplements as prescribed.
   c. Do not take additional vitamins without your physician's approval.
3. *Information on medicine used to treat colitis and related disorders*
   a. If you have been prescribed sulfasalazine (Azulfidine), be sure to eat rich food sources of folic acid, such as dark green vegetables, every day. If you tend to get diarrhea when you eat vegetables, you can eat fortified breakfast cereal, which is a good source of folic acid. The medicine you are taking increases your need for this vitamin.
4. *Information on medicine used to treat constipation*
   a. Laxatives are rarely necessary and you should take them only when they are prescribed by a physician.
   b. The best ways to avoid constipation are
      - Drink plenty of water.
      - Eat high-fiber foods, such as bran-containing breakfast cereals.
      - Drink a hot beverage with your breakfast.
      - Take regular, daily exercise.
   c. All laxatives, other than stool softeners, can deprive your body of potassium, which can lead to severe muscle weakness.
   d. Avoid regular, daily use of mineral oil, since it can prevent absorption of the fat-soluble vitamins in your food, including vitamin A, vitamin D, and vitamin K.

E. *For patients with endocrine diseases*
   1. *Information for patients with diabetes taking insulin*

a. Be sure to eat regularly and promptly after injecting your insulin. Maintain a constant dietary pattern, following the instructions you have been given on your diabetes diet.
b. Be sure to eat a bedtime snack, as advised by your physician.
c. Check your blood sugar each day, at the times indicated by your physician, and record the blood sugar levels. Report these levels to your physician; telephone your physician if your blood sugar is either above or below the acceptable limits.
d. If you go to a new physician for another health problem, be sure to tell this physician about your current diabetes treatment.
e. Do not take over-the-counter medication; in particular, do not take cold medicines containing ephedrine or similar drugs. They can raise your blood sugar.
f. If you plan to be away from home and are likely to miss a meal, carry a piece of fruit, some raisins, or fruit juice with you so that you do not become hypoglycemic.
g. Report infections, including minor infections such as boils and dental abscesses, to your physician. They can lead to serious loss of diabetes control.
h. If you plan to begin a new form of physical exercise, discuss it with your physician so that your insulin dose can be adjusted as necessary to prevent undue lowering of your blood sugar.

2. *Information to patients with diabetes taking oral agents*
   a. Take your diabetes pills every day at same time(s) you have been instructed to take them. For the short-acting agents such as glipizide, the best time to take the morning dose is on waking and approximately 1/2 to 1 hour before breakfast.
   b. If you are taking oral antidiabetic medications, it is best to avoid drinking alcohol. If you are taking chlorpropamide (Diabinese), you may flush unpleasantly if you drink any alcohol.
   c. Measure your blood sugar regularly and report both high and low values to your physician.
   d. If you are taking a long-acting oral agent, eat a bedtime snack as directed to avoid excessive lowering of your blood sugar.

e. Follow your diabetes diet, which should help you restrict your calorie and fat consumption and lose the necessary weight. Weigh yourself every week, and keep a record of your weight.
f. Be sure to explain to all physicians you see that you have diabetes. Otherwise, they might prescribe medications that cause loss of diabetes control. The most important of these are cortisone-like medicines, thiazide diuretics, cold medicines (which can elevate your blood sugar), sulfa drugs, aspirin-containing drugs, and certain blood pressure medicine such as propranolol (Inderal), which can lower your blood sugar to a point that you can become hypoglycemic.

F. *For patients with arthritis*

1. *Information on medicines used to control rheumatoid arthritis*
   a. If you are taking a cortisone-like medication such as prednisone, you are at risk for bone thinning (osteoporosis). You should discuss this with your physician, who will advise you how much calcium you should be getting from dairy foods. He or she may also advise you to take calcium pills to lower the risk of bone problems.
   b. If you are taking penicillamine (Cuprimine), you may experience loss of taste or appetite, which are side effects of the drug. If you do, report it to your physician.
   c. If you take penicillamine, it is advisable to take a multivitamin-mineral supplement because the medication can increase your need for vitamin B_6 and zinc.
   d. If you are taking methotrexate, have your blood checked regularly for anemia and report any weight loss to your physician.
2. *Information on medicine used to control osteoarthritis*
   a. If you are taking one or more antiarthritis medications of the ibuprofen type daily, you may experience side effects that lead to acute and long-term health and nutritional problems.
      - Acute problems include swelling of your legs and feet, loss of appetite, nausea, gas, and stomach ache. You may also vomit and bring up blood or pass blood in your bowel movement. Bowel movement containing blood may not be easily recognized. It may be black, rather than covered with fresh blood.

- Longer-term side effects include anemia and severe loss of kidney function. Before such kidney function changes occur, the level of potassium in your blood may increase.

b. The risk factors for developing anemia while you are taking antiarthritis medicine are
   - A previous history of gastric or duodenal ulcer
   - Heavy use of alcohol and intake of a diet that is very low in iron. Such diets often contain no meats or fish or are very low in calories.

c. Risk factors for high potassium levels in your blood while you are taking one of these antiarthritis medications include
   - Taking potassium-sparing diuretics
   - Taking potassium supplements
   - Using salt substitutes

d. Risk factors for kidney disease while you are taking these medications include
   - High doses of the antiarthritis medications
   - Diabetes

e. To avoid the side effects of antiarthritis medicine or to achieve an early and complete recovery from the side effects, take the following precautions
   - Tell the physician who prescribes the antiarthritis medicine what other medications you are taking.
   - Never take potassium supplements when the need no longer exists—that is, when you are taking a diuretic that does not deprive your body of potassium.
   - Report all signs of indigestion and all evidence of stomach or intestinal bleeding to your physician.
   - Ask your physician to check your blood for anemia at least once a month, have your potassium level taken, and have lab tests for kidney function.

3. *Information on medicine used to treat gout*

   a. If you are taking colchicine, you may experience diarrhea and pass large, pale-colored stools that float in the toilet bowl. This change in your bowel movements means that the colchicine is keeping you from absorbing your food properly. This effect of the medicine, though unpleasant, may not do you serious harm unless you continue taking the colchicine for more than 10 days at a time. Find out from your physician how long you should be taking the medicine.

b. If you are prescribed allopurinol and you are already taking a medicine to thin your blood or prevent blood clots (an anticoagulant), you need to have blood tests taken at regular intervals, usually weekly, to measure your "pro time" (prothrombin time). Allopurinol increases the duration of action of these blood thinners, and that can increase your risk of bleeding.

G. *For patients with neurological or psychiatric problems*

1. *Information on medicine used for the control of seizures*

a. If you are prescribed phenytoin (Dilantin) or phenobarbital, your needs for certain vitamins are increased. You particularly have a greater need for the B vitamin, folic acid. You can meet this need by increasing your intake of dark green vegetables like broccoli and spinach and of fortified breakfast foods. Do not take B vitamin supplements unless they are prescribed by your physician, because too much folic acid or vitamin B_6 can interfere with seizure control.

b. If you are taking phenytoin or phenobarbital, you have an increased need for vitamin D. If you are not able to get outdoors so that the sunshine can make vitamin D in your skin, you must either increase your intake of dairy foods (particularly milk) or take a vitamin D supplement. Discuss your need for vitamin D with your physician and ask how much you should take. Do not self-medicate with vitamin D, because too high a dose of this vitamin can cause kidney damage.

2. *Information on medicine used for the control of Parkinson's disease*

a. If you are prescribed a medication containing levodopa (eg, Sinemet), you should take the medicine with food to avoid gastric irritation. However, do not take it with meat, meat extracts, fish, or other high-protein foods, or with liquid formula supplements.

b. Do not take supplements of vitamin B_6 if you are taking a medication with levodopa. A high intake of vitamin B_6 from supplements can interfere with the effectiveness of the medication in the control of your Parkinson's disease.

c. If you are taking amantadine (Symmetrel) or benztropine (Cogentin), your mouth may tend to get very dry. It will be easier for you to swallow solid food if you drink water or another beverage at the same time.

3. *Information on medicines used for the control of manic states and depression*

   a. If you are taking lithium, do not alter your salt intake without consulting with your physician. Too little salt in your diet can increase the risk of side effects from the lithium (such as water retention, mental confusion, and kidney problems). Eating too many high-salt foods, like olives, salted nuts, or cold cuts, can prevent the lithium from working properly. In addition, if you go to a new physician and he or she says you need blood pressure medicine, be sure to mention that you are taking lithium so you will not be given a diuretic that takes sodium out of your body.

   b. If you are given an antidepressant called phenelzine or a related medication, you must not eat aged cheese or drink wine or beer. Those foods might cause a dangerous increase in your blood pressure. If you are given an antidepressant, it is best to ask your physician which one you have been given.

4. *Information on medicine used for the control of abnormal behavior other than depression*

   If you have been prescribed a tranquilizer like chlorpromazine (Thorazine) or thioridazine (Mellaril), you may experience a large increase in your appetite. If this happens, talk to a dietitian, who can explain how you can overcome your hunger by eating low-calorie foods. If you do not get such help, you may gain too much weight.

5. *Information on disulfiram (Antabuse), used to control alcohol abuse*

   a. If you have been prescribed disulfiram, you must avoid alcoholic beverages and foods containing wine or liquor totally. Drinking any alcohol at all will cause a severe reaction: you will get a terrible headache and/or pains in your chest, and you will get sick to your stomach.

   b. While you are taking disulfiram, you must also avoid all

medications containing alcohol, including over-the-counter cough medicines and tonics.

H. *For patients with chronic, noninfective skin diseases*

a. If you are taking isotretinoin (Accutane) for acne, you should avoid a high-fat diet, since this medication can increase the fat content (triglyceride level) of your blood.

b. Isotretinoin can also increase blood sugar levels. Your plasma cholesterol, plasma triglycerides, and blood glucose levels should be checked every month.

c. Side effects of the medicine are similar to those from vitamin A, including dry skin, dry eyes, ache in the neck, upper back pain, and reduced liver function. Taking vitamin A with isotretinoin increases the risk of side effects due to the medication.

d. Isotretinoin taken during the first trimester of pregnancy can cause birth defects and growth retardation in the fetus.

I. *For patients taking medicine for protozoal and fungal infections*

a. If you are taking metronidazole (Flagyl) to control either *Giardia* infections or trichomonal vaginal infections, you should avoid all alcoholic beverages. Drinking alcohol can cause nausea, vomiting, and headache.

b. If you are taking a medication that contains the drug pyrimethamine (such as Fansidar) to prevent or treat malaria, you are at risk for folate deficiency. Ask your physician if you should take a folic acid supplement.

c. If you are taking griseofulvin to control athlete's foot or another fungal infection, take it with or immediately after the evening meal. The fat in the meal promotes absorption of the medication. Do not drink alcoholic beverages, because they may give you a severe headache.

d. If you are taking ketoconazole for a fungal infection, remember that nausea after a meal may be a sign of serious side effects on your liver. Report any such nausea to your physician. Women who are breastfeeding should not take ketoconazole, because it gets into breast milk and can harm the baby.

J. *For patients taking medicine for urinary infections*

a. If you are taking methenamine (Mandelamine) to control a urinary infection, drink a glass of cranberry juice before each dose. The juice may help to acidify your urine, which will aid the action of the medication.

b. If you are taking nitrofurantoin (Furadantin) for a urinary infection, it is best to take it after eating to reduce the risk of stomach irritation.

K. *For women taking oral contraceptives*

a. Women who take oral contraceptives have slightly increased needs for certain B vitamins, including folic acid and vitamin B_6. These increased needs can be satisfied by a good intake of these vitamins in your diet. Good food sources of folic acid are dark green vegetables. Good food sources of vitamin B_6 are meats, whole grain cereals, and nuts. Do not take megadoses of vitamin B_6, because they can cause nerve damage.

GENERAL REFERENCES FOR PATIENTS ON PREVENTION OF DRUG AND NUTRIENT INTERACTIONS

1. *About Your Medicines.* US Pharmacopeial Convention Inc, 12601 Twinbrook Parkway, Rockville, MD 20852, updated annually.
2. Pronsky, ZM. *Powers & Moore's Food Medication Interactions.* 8th ed. Pottstown, PA: Ford-Medication Interactions, 1993.
3. Nutrition Screening Initiative. *Nutrition Interventions Manual for Professionals Caring for Older Americans.* Washington, DC: Greer, Margolis, Mitchell, Grunwald & Associates, Inc., 1992.

Appendix

D Glossary of Terms

ACE-I angiotensin I-converting enzyme inhibitor
Anorexia loss of appetite
Antifolate folate antagonist
Aplastic anemia anemia associated with suppression of bone marrow function

BP blood pressure
Bronchodilator drug used to dilute tubes in air passages
Bulimia bout of excessive eating followed by vomiting

Ca++ calcium
CBC complete blood count
Chol cholesterol
CK check

Diabetogenic drug drug causing elevation of blood sugar
Disulfiram reaction acute reaction with nausea, vomiting, and chest pain occurring when alcohol is taken with certain other drugs (eg, Antabuse)

Effective dose the dosage of a drug that may be expected to cause a specific intensity of effect (*Mosby's Medical Dictionary*)
EGR erythrocyte glutathione reductase
Enteropathy condition of small intestine usually associated with impaired absorption of nutrients

Facts & Comparisons drug manual used by pharmacists
Fe iron

G6PD glucose-6-phosphate dehydrogenase

Glycemia control control of blood sugar in diabetes

H2 receptor antagonist drug that suppresses acid production in the stomach

Hyperglycemia high blood sugar

Hyperkalemia high plasma or serum potassium

Hypoalbuminemia low plasma or serum albumin (reflects protein-energy malnutrition)

Hypocalcemia low plasma or serum calcemia

Hypoglycemia low blood sugar

Hypokalemia low plasma or serum potassium

Hypomagnesemia low plasma or serum magnesium

Hyponatremia low plasma or serum sodium

K+ potassium

Kcal kilocalories

Loop diuretic diuretic affecting loop of Henle in the kidney

MAOI monoamine oxidase inhibitor

Megaloblastosis enlargement of red blood cells associated with maturation defect found in vitamin B_2 or folate deficiency

Mg++ magnesium

Na+ sodium

Neuropathy disorder of peripheral or autonomic nerves

NSAID nonsteroidal antiinflammatory drug

Osteomalacia condition of vitamin D deficiency in an adult

PEM protein energy malnutrition

Protime prothrombin time

Pyridoxine vitamin B_6

Riboflavin vitamin B_2

Tartrazine yellow dye #5

Thiazide type of diuretic

Triglyceride plasma or serum level of fat

Tyramine reaction acute elevation of blood pressure occurring when foods containing the amine tyramine (such as aged cheese) are eaten when drugs are being taken that are in a category known to inhibit amine degradation

USPDI U.S. Pharmacopeia drug information

Appendix

E

Acceptable Values for Blood Levels of Nutrients in SI Units and Drug-Related Reasons for Monitoring

NUTRIENT	ACCEPTABLE VALUES SI UNITS	POTENTIAL EFFECT OF DRUGS
Folate	4-22 nmol/L	Drugs that may reduce level include methotrexate, alcohol, oral contraceptives, aspirin, and phenytoin.
25-OH vitamin D_3	45-90 nmol/L	Drugs that may reduce levels include phenytoin and isoniazid.
Vitamin B_{12}	150-750 pmol/L	Drugs that may reduce level include cimetidine and related drugs taken for more than 6 months.
Sodium	135-147 nmol/L	Diuretics may reduce levels; also chlorpromazine.
Potassium	3.5-5.0 nmol/L	Diuretics may reduce levels.
Magnesium	0.8-1.2 mmol/L	Diuretics and cisplatin may reduce levels.
Calcium	male 2.20-2.58 mmol/L female < 50 yrs 2.20-2.50 mmol/L > 50 yrs 2.20-2.56 mmol/L	Drugs that may reduce level include isoniazid, phenytoin, and rifampin. Drugs that may increase level include tamoxifen, calcium carbonate, and sodium bicarbonate.
Creatinine	50-110 μmol/L	Drugs that may increase level include NSAIDs, procainamide, amphoterian B, and sodium bicarbonate.

REFERENCE

Young DS. Implementation of SI units for clinical laboratory values. *Ann Intern Med*. 1987;106:114-129.

Appendix

F

Monitoring Drug Therapy: Guide to Therapeutic Drug Levels and Reason for Monitoring Change in Levels with New Diet Prescriptions or ADR

DRUG	THERAPEUTIC DRUG LEVEL	REASON FOR MONITORING
Digoxin	1.0-2.6 nmol/L	Plasma needs to be <2.0 nmol/L level if hypokalemia is present.
Lithium carbonate	0.4-0.8 mmol/L	Increase in sodium intake level leads to reduction in drug level and loss of drug effect. Reduction in salt intake leads to increase in drug and risk of toxicity.
Phenytoin	40-80 mcgmol/L	Increase in folic acid intake to 5 mg/day or greater can lead to reduction in plasma level and loss of seizure control.
Theophylline	50-110 mcgmol/L	Increase in protein level of the diet leads to decrease in drug level to below therapeutic range. Meals high in fat lead to rapid increase in plasma level and acute toxicity.

REFERENCES

Aronson JK, Hardman M. Digoxin. *Br Med J.* 1992;305:1149.

Aronson JK, Reynolds DJM. Lithium. *Br Med J.* 1992;305:1273-1276.

Roe DA. *Diet and Drug Interactions.* New York: Van Nostrand Reinhold: 1989: 21.

Aronson JK, Hardman M, Reynolds, DJM. Phenytoin. *Br Med J.* 1992;305:1215-1217.

Appendix

G

Patient Instructions on Benefits, Risks, and Safe Usage of High-Dose Vitamin and Mineral Supplements

VITAMIN/ MINERAL	BENEFITS	RISKS	SAFE USAGE	REF.
Beta-carotene	Can protect against some types of light sensitivity.	Yellowing of the skin.	Must be taken daily.	1
	Prevents loss of immune function due to UV light exposure.			2
	May reduce cancer risk.			
	Safe precursor of vitamin A.			3
Vitamin A	High-dose supplements are not required.	Can cause liver damage, bone defects, hair loss, headaches, and birth defects.	Should not be taken in amounts exceeding the RDA.	4-8
Vitamin D	Topical treatment with vitamin D derivative, calciprotriol, clears psoriasis.	Causes high blood pressure.	Vitamin D supplements above the RDA should not be taken, except when ordered by an MD.	9, 10

VITAMIN/ MINERAL	BENEFITS	RISKS	SAFE USAGE	REF.
Vitamin E	Can improve immunity.	May cause bleeding in those taking drugs to prevent blood clots (eg, warfarin).	Should not be taken by people on warfarin or related anti-coagulants.	11, 12
Vitamin K	Prevents excessive bleeding from anti-coagulants. Long-term, broad-spectrum antibiotics.	May lessen efficacy of drugs like warfarin.	Should not be taken by people on warfarin or related anti-coagulants.	13
Thiamin	High doses (200 mg bid) iv should be given to alcoholics to treat Wernicke's enceph-alopathy.	Can cause allergic reactions.	Should be given by an MD in a hospital setting.	14, 15
Riboflavin	High doses are required to treat acute borate poisoning. Dose is 5-10 mg tid orally.	Can cause risk of phototoxic reactions due to drugs (if given iv).	Should be given by an MD in a hospital setting.	16

VITAMIN/ MINERAL	BENEFITS	RISKS	SAFE USAGE	REF.
Niacin	High doses reduce blood cholesterol.	Causes flushing. Risks of long-term use are damage to liver, thyroid, and bone marrow. Can cause syncope if taken with beta-adrenergic blocking drugs.	Doses greater than the RDA should only be taken when advised by an MD. Can increase blood glucose.	17-20
Vitamin B_6	Required if taking the anti-Tb drug isoniazid, or the anti-hypertensive drug hydralazine or oral contraceptives.	Can cause nerve damage.	Should only be taken if ordered by an MD.	21-24
Folic acid	Can reduce the risk of bearing infant with neural tube defect in women with previous history, if taken at least 1 mo prior to pregnancy and through early pregnancy.	Can reduce absorption of antiseizure Rx if >15 mg/day is given.	Should be taken as prescribed by MD.	25,26

VITAMIN/ MINERAL	BENEFITS	RISKS	SAFE USAGE	REF.
	Can reduce the risk of toxicity due to low-dose methotrexate for rheumatoid arthritis. The dose is 1 mg/day.	>1 mg/day can mask lab test for vitamin B_{12} deficiency.		26-28
Vitamin C	May decrease the risk of cataracts and of stomach cancer.	Can cause proctitis and diarrhea; also renal calculi.	Should not be taken by patients with hyperoxaluria.	29,30, 31
Calcium	Can reduce the risk of osteoporosis.	Interferes with the absorption of tetracycline.*	Should not be taken within 2 hrs of taking this antibiotic.	32

*Iron supplements also interfere with the absorption of tetracycline.

REFERENCES

1. Mathews-Roth MN. Carotenoid functions in photoprotection and cancer prevention. *J Environ Pathol Topical Oncol.* 1990;10:181-192.
2. Fuller CJ, Faulkner H, Bendich A, Parker RS, Roe DA. Effect of beta carotene supplementation on photosuppression of delayed type hypersensitivity in young men. *Am J Clin Nutr.* 1992;56:684-690.
3. Bendich A. Safety issues regarding use of vitamin supplements. In: Sauberlich HE, Machlin LJ, eds. *Beyond Deficiency: New Views on the Function and Health Effects of Vitamins. Ann NY Acad Sci.* 1992;669:300-312.
4. Muenter, Perry HO, Ludwig J. Chronic vitamin A intoxication in adults. *Am J Med.* 1971;30:1291-1294.
5. Hatoff DE, Gertler SL, Miyal K, Parker BA, Weiss JB. Hypervitaminosis A unmasked by acute viral hepatitis. *Gastroenterology.* 1982;82:124-128.
6. Frame B, Jackson CE, Reynolds WA, Umphrey JE. Hypercalcemia and skeletal effects of chronic hypervitaminosis A. *Ann Intern Med.* 1974;80:44-48.

7. Roe DA. *Diet and Drug Interactions.* New York: Van Nostrand Reinhold; 1989:113-115.
8. Lammer EJ, Chen DT, Hoar RM, Agnish ND, Benke PJ, Braun JT, Curry CJ, Fernhoff PM, Grix AW, Lott LT, Richard JM, Sun SC. Retinoic acid embryopathy. *N Engl J Med.* 1985;313:837-841.
9. Taussig HB. Possible injury to the cardiovascular system from vitamin D. *Ann Intern Med.* 1966;65:1195-1197.
10. Menne T, Larsen K. Psoriasis treatment with vitamin D derivatives. *Semin Dermatol.* 1992;11:278-283.
11. Meydani SN, Barklund MP, Liu S, Meydani M, Miller RA, Cannon JG, Morrow FD, Rocklin R, Blumberg JB. Vitamin E supplementation enhances cell-mediated immunity in healthy elderly subjects. *Am J Clin Nutr.* 1990; 52:557-563.
12. Corrigan JJ Jr, Marcus FI. Coagulopathy associated with vitamin E ingestion. *JAMA.* 1974;230:1300-1301.
13. Lee M, Schwartz RN, Sharifi R. Warfarin resistance and vitamin K. *Arch Intern Med.* 1981;94:140-141.
14. Greengard P. The water-soluble vitamins. In: Goodman LS, Gilman A, eds. *The Pharmacological Basis of Therapeutics.* 5th ed. New York: Macmillan Publ; 1975:1550.
15. Roe DA. *Alcohol and the Diet.* Westport, Conn: AVI Publ Co; 1979:126-131.
16. Roe DA. *Diet and Drug Interactions.* 1989:1.
17. Canner PL, Berge KG, Wenger NK, et al. Fifteen-year mortality in coronary drug project patients: long-term benefits from niacin. *J Am Coll Cardiol.* 1986;8:1245-1255.
18. Goldstein MR. Potential problems with the widespread use of niacin. *Am J Med.* 1988;85:881.
19. O'Brien T, Silverberg JD, Nguyen TT. Nicotinic acid-induced toxicity associated with cytopenia and decreased levels of thyroxine-binding globulin. *Mayo Clin Proc.* 1992;67:465-468.
20. *Drug Facts and Comparisons.* St Louis, MO: Facts and Comparisons; 1992: 19.
21. Brown CV. Acute isoniazid poisoning. *Ann Rev Resp Dis.* 1972;105:206-216.
22. Roe DA. *Alcohol and the Diet.* 1979:126-131.
23. Schaumberg H, Kaplan HJ, Windebank A, Vick N, Rasmus S, Pleasure D, Brown MJ. Sensory neuropathy from pyridoxine abuse: a new megavitamin syndrome. *N Engl J Med.* 1983;309:445-448.
24. Raskin NH, Fishman RA. Peridoxine-deficiency neuropathy due to hydralazine. *N Engl J Med.* 1965;273:1182-1185.
25. Recommendations for the use of folic acid to reduce the number of cases of spina bifida and other neural tube defects. *MMWR.* 1992;41:1-7.
26. Butterworth CE, Tamura T. Folic acid safety and toxicity: a brief review. *Am J Clin Nutr.* 1989;50:353-358.

27. Chanarin I, Deacon R, Lumb M, Perry J. Cobalamin and folate: recent developments. *J Clin Pathol.* 1992;45:277-283.
28. Morgan SL, Baggott JE, Vaughn WH, Young PK, Austin JV, Krumdieck CL, Alarcon GS. The effect of folic acid supplementation on the toxicity of low-dose methotrexate in patients with rheumatoid arthritis. *Arthrit Rheum.* 1990;33:9-18.
29. Jacques PF, Hartz SC, Chylack LT, McGandy RB, Sadowski JA. Nutritional status in persons with and without senile cataract: blood vitamin and mineral levels. *Am J Clin Nutr.* 1988;48:152-158.
30. Briggs MH, Garcia Webb P, Davies P. Urinary oxalate and vitamin C supplements. *Lancet.* 1973;2:201.
31. Korner WF, Weber P. Tolerance of high ascorbic acid doses. *Int J Vit Res.* 1972;42:528-530.
32. Gibaldi M. *Biopharmaceutics and Clinical Pharmacokinetics.* 2nd ed. Philadelphia: Lea & Febiger; 1977:27-65.

Indexes

Disease Index

VIII. NEOPLASTIC

VIII.1	Leukemia, Hodgkin's disease, and cancer	Antiestrogenics	76
		Anti-Hodgkin's	73
		Antineoplastics	74–75
		Narcotic analgesics	76

VI. NEUROLOGICAL AND PSYCHIATRIC

VI.5	Alcoholism	Alcohol aversion drugs	62
		Laxative/antiliver failure	63
VI.4	Dementias and paranoid states	Antianxieties	62
		Antipsychotics and antiemetics	60–61
		Anti-TIAs	62
VI.3	Manic-depressive psychosis and other depressive states	Antianxieties	59
		Antidepressants	58–59
		Antiinsomnias	59
		Antimania	58
		Stimulants	59
VI.2	Parkinson's disease	Anticholinergics	57
		Anti-Parkinson	55–56
		Dopamine receptor agonists	57
		Dopaminergics	57
VI.1	Seizure disorders	Anticonvulsants	51–53

II. RESPIRATORY

II.1	Asthma	Antiallergics	21
		Bronchodilators	17–20
		Expectorants	21
		Glucocorticoids	20
II.2	Bronchitis and pneumonia	Antibacterials	23
		Antibiotics	22,23
II.3	Tuberculosis	Antituberculosis	24–25

Problem Index

PROBLEM	DRUG CAUSING PROBLEM	DISEASE PRESENT IF THIS DRUG IS TAKEN	PAGE
Anemia	Amphotericin B	AIDS; fungal infection	80,84
	Aspirin	Rheumatoid arthritis	44
	Azidothymidine	AIDS	79
	Carbamazepine	Seizure disorder	53
	Chloroquine HCI	Malaria	83
	Diflunisal	Osteoarthritis	45
	Fenoprofen	Osteoarthritis	45
	Ibuprofen†	Osteoarthritis	45
	Indomethacin	Osteoarthritis	45
	Ketoprofen	Osteoarthritis	45
	Meclofenamate	Osteoarthritis	45
	Methotrexate	Rheumatoid arthritis; cancer	43,75
	Naproxen	Osteoarthritis	45
	Phenobarbital	Seizure disorder	52
	Phenytoin	Seizure disorder	51
	Piroxicam	Osteoarthritis	45
	Primidone	Seizure disorder	53
	Probucol	Atherosclerosis	6
	Pyrazinamide	Tuberculosis	25
	Pyrimethamine	Malaria	82
	Sulfadoxine and pyrimethamine	Malaria	82
	Sulindac	Osteoarthritis	46
	Tolmetin	Osteoarthritis	46
	Trimethoprim	Bronchitis; pneumonia	23
	Trimetrexate	Cancer	75
	Valproic acid	Seizure disorder	53
Anorexia	Amiloride	Heart disease	2
	Amiodarone	Heart disease	3

PROBLEM	DRUG CAUSING PROBLEM	DISEASE PRESENT IF THIS DRUG IS TAKEN	PAGE
	Amphotericin B	AIDS	80
	Azidothymidine	AIDS	79
	Bromocriptine	Parkinson's disease	57
	Captopril	Hypertension	7
	Carbamazepine	Seizure disorder	53
	Carbidopa and levodopa	Parkinson's disease	56
	Digoxin	Heart disease	1
	Enalapril	Hypertension	8
	Encainide	Heart disease	2
	Etretinate	Psoriasis	69
	5-Fluorouracil	Cancer	74
	Gemfibrozil	Atherosclerosis	6
	Levodopa	Parkinson's disease	55
	Methotrexate	Cancer	75
	Morphine	Cancer	76
	Omeprazole	Peptic ulcer	30
	Penicillamine	Rheumatoid arthritis	43
	Pentamidine	AIDS	79
	Pentoxifylline	Thrombosis; psychosis	5,62
	Probucol	Atherosclerosis	6
	Procainamide	Heart disease	2
	Rauwolfia	Hypertension	9
	Theophylline	Asthma	17
Bleeding	Cefamandole	Bronchitis; pneumonia	22
	Cefoperazone	Bronchitis; pneumonia	22
	Cefotetan	Bronchitis; pneumonia	22
	Cimetidine	Peptic ulcer	29

PROBLEM	DRUG CAUSING PROBLEM	DISEASE PRESENT IF THIS DRUG IS TAKEN	PAGE
	Moxalactam	Bronchitis; pneumonia	22
	Phenobarbital	Seizure disorder	52
	Phenytoin	Seizure disorder	51
	Ranitidine	Peptic ulcer	30
	Valproic acid	Seizure disorder	53
	Warfarin	Thrombosis	4
Constipation	Amantadine	Parkinson's disease	57
	Benztropine	Parkinson's disease	57
	Cholestyramine	Atherosclerosis	5
	Colestipol	Atherosclerosis	6
	Haloperidol	Psychosis	61
	Morphine	Cancer	76
	Sulfalfate	Peptic ulcer	32
	Vincristine	Cancer	75
Diarrhea	Amphotericin B	AIDS	80
	Azithromycin	Bronchitis; pneumonia	22
	Cyclophosphamide	Cancer	74
	Dactinomycin	Cancer	74
	Erythromycin	Bronchitis; pneumonia	22
	Etretinate	Psoriasis	69
	5-Fluorouracil	Cancer	74
	Fluconazole	AIDS	80
	Methotrexate	Cancer	75
	Misoprostol	Peptic ulcer	30
	Nitrofurantoin	Urinary infection	87
	Olsalzine	Inflammatory bowel disease	34
	Vincristine	Cancer	75
Disulfiram reaction	Disulfiram	Alcoholism	62
	Metronidazole	Giardiasis	81
Dry mouth	Amantadine	Parkinson's disease	57

PROBLEM	DRUG CAUSING PROBLEM	DISEASE PRESENT IF THIS DRUG IS TAKEN	PAGE
	Benztropine	Parkinson's disease	57
	Captopril	Hypertension	7
	Clonidine	Hypertension	8
	Diazepam	Psychosis	62
	Diphenoxylate with atropine	Inflammatory bowel disease	35
	Enalapril	Hypertension	7
	Gemfibrozil	Atherosclerosis	6
	Guanabenz	Hypertension	9
	Haloperidol	Psychosis	61
	Methyldopa	Hypertension	8
	Omeprazole	Peptic ulcer	30
	Pentoxifylline	Thrombosis	5
	Propantheline	Peptic ulcer	32
Flush	Alcohol in cough medicine	Bronchitis	21
	Chlorpropamide	Diabetes	39
	Griseofulvin	Fungal infection	83
	Iodinated glycerol	Asthma	21
	Niacin	Atherosclerosis	6
	Nifedipine	Hypertension	11
	Potassium iodide	Asthma	21
	Theophylline	Asthma	17
Folate deficiency	Cholestyramine	Atherosclerosis	5
	Colestipol	Atherosclerosis	6
	Methotrexate	Rheumatoid arthritis; cancer	43,75
	Pentamidine	AIDS	79
	Phenobarbital	Seizure disorder	52
	Phenytoin	Seizure disorder	51
	Primidone	Seizure disorder	53
	Pyrimethamine	Malaria	82
	Sulfadoxine and pyrimethamine	Malaria	82

PROBLEM	DRUG CAUSING PROBLEM	DISEASE PRESENT IF THIS DRUG IS TAKEN	PAGE
	Sulfasalazine	Inflammatory bowel disease	34
	Triamterene	Heart disease	2
	Trimethoprim	Bronchitis; pneumonia	23
	Trimetrexate	Cancer	75
Gout	Cyclosporine	Psoriasis	70
	Ethambutol	Tuberculosis	26
	Hydrochlorothiazide	Hypertension	10
	Thiazides	Hypertension	10
Hemorrhage	Warfarin*	Thromphlebitis	41
	Warfarin and allopurinol	Thrombophlebitis and gout	46
	Warfarin and clofibrate	Thrombophlebitis and atherosclerosis	6
	Warfarin and levothyroxine	Thrombophlebitis and myxedema (or thyroid hypo-function)	41
	Warfarin and propylthiouracil	Thrombophlebitis and myxedema	41
Hypercalcemia	Pentamidine	AIDS	79
	Sodium bicarbonate and milk diet	Peptic ulcer	30
	Tamoxifen	Cancer	76
Hyperglycemia	Albuterol	Asthma	19
	Encainide	Heart disease	2
	Niacin	Atherosclerosis	6
	Orasone	Asthma	20
	Prednisone	Asthma; rheumatoid arthritis	20,43
	Thiazides	Hypertension	10
Hyperkalemia	Amiloride	Heart disease	2

PROBLEM	DRUG CAUSING PROBLEM	DISEASE PRESENT IF THIS DRUG IS TAKEN	PAGE
	Captopril	Hypertension	7
	Diflunisal	Osteoarthritis	45
	Enalapril	Hypertension	8
	Fenoprofen	Osteoarthritis	45
	Ibuprofen†	Osteoarthritis	45
	Indomethacin	Osteoarthritis	45
	Ketoprofen	Osteoarthritis	45
	Meclofenamate	Osteoarthritis	45
	Naproxen	Osteoarthritis	45
	Piroxicam	Osteoarthritis	45
	Potassium iodide	Asthma	21
	Spironolactone	Heart disease	2
	Sulindac	Osteoarthritis	46
	Tolmetin	Osteoarthritis	46
	Triamterene	Heart disease	2
Hypoglycemia	Atenolol	Hypertension	10
	Chlorpropamide	Diabetes	39
	Glyburide	Diabetes	40
	Insulin	Diabetes	39
	Metoprolol	Hypertension	9
	Nadolol	Hypertension	10
	Propranolol	Hypertension	9
	Sulfadoxine and pyrimethamine	Malaria	82
	Timolol	Hypertension	10
Hypokalemia	Amphotericin B	Fungal infection	84
	Bumetanide	Heart disease	2
	Carbidopa and levodopa	Parkinson's disease	56
	Ethacrynic acid	Heart disease	2
	Furosemide	Heart disease	1
	Hydrochlorothiazide	Hypertension	10
	Levodopa	Parkinson's disease	56
	Thiazides	Hypertension	10

PROBLEM	DRUG CAUSING PROBLEM	DISEASE PRESENT IF THIS DRUG IS TAKEN	PAGE
Hyponatremia	Amiloride	Heart disease	2
	Bumetanide	Heart disease	2
	Chlorpromazine	Psychosis	60
	Ethacrynic acid	Heart disease	2
	Fluphenazine	Psychosis	61
	Furosemide	Heart disease	1
	Hydrochlorothiazide	Hypertension	10
	Perphenazine	Psychosis	61
	Spironolactone	Heart disease	2
	Thioridazine	Psychosis	61
	Vincristine	Cancer	75
Lithium toxicity	Lithium	Psychosis	58
Nausea/ vomiting	Amiodarone	Heart disease	3
	Amphotericin B	AIDS	80
	Azidothymidine	AIDS	79
	Azithromycin	Bronchitis; pneumonia	22
	Bleomycin	Cancer	74
	Bromocriptine	Parkinson's disease	57
	Captopril	Hypertension	7
	Clofibrate	Atherosclerosis	6
	Cromolyn	Asthma	21
	Cyclophosphatamide	Cancer	74
	Dactinomycin	Cancer	74
	Digoxin	Heart disease	1
	Disulfiram	Alcoholism	62
	Enalapril	Hypertension	8
	Encainide	Heart disease	2
	Erythromycin	Bronchitis; pneumonia	22
	Ethambutol	Tuberculosis	25
	5-Fluorouracil	Cancer	74
	Fluconazole	AIDS	80
	Ketoconazole	Fungal infection	83

PROBLEM	DRUG CAUSING PROBLEM	DISEASE PRESENT IF THIS DRUG IS TAKEN	PAGE
	Lomustine	Cancer	75
	Methyldopa	Hypertension	8
	Metoclopramide	Peptic ulcer	32
	Metronidazole	Giardiasis	81
	Misoprostol	Peptic ulcer	30
	Pentamidine	AIDS	79
	Pentoxifylline	Psychosis	62
	Pentoxitylline	Thrombosis	5
	Procainamide	Heart disease	2
	Vincristine	Cancer	75
Osteoporosis	Prednisone[‡]	Asthma; inflammatory bowel disease; rheumatoid arthritis	20,34,43
Sore mouth	Carbamazepine	Seizure disorder	53
	Bleomycin	Cancer	74
	Vincristine	Cancer	75
Stomatitis	Dactinomycin	Rheumatoid arthritis	74
	5-Fluorouracil	Cancer	74
	Methotrexate	Rheumatoid arthritis; cancer	43,75
	Sulfadoxine and pyrimethamine	Malaria	82
Sulfite reaction	Isoetharine	Asthma	20
Tartrazine reaction	Carbidopa and levodopa	Parkinson's disease	56
	Hydralazine	Hypertension	8
	Levodopa	Parkinson's disease	55
	Methenamine	Urinary infection	87
	Sulindac	Osteoarthritis	46
Tyramine reaction	Carbidopa and levodopa	Parkinson's disease	56
	Levodopa	Parkinson's disease	55
	Phenelzine	Depression	58
	Procarbazine	Hodgkin's disease	73

PROBLEM	DRUG CAUSING PROBLEM	DISEASE PRESENT IF THIS DRUG IS TAKEN	PAGE
Vitamin B_6 deficiency	Carbidopa and levodopa	Parkinson's disease	56
	Hydralazine	Hypertension	8
	Isoniazid	Tuberculosis	24
	Levodopa	Parkinson's disease	55
	Penicillamine	Arthritis	43
	Pyrazinamide	Tuberculosis	25
Vitamin B_{12} deficiency	Cholestyramine	Atherosclerosis	5
	Cimetidine	Peptic ulcer	29
	Famotidine	Peptic ulcer	30
	Ranitidine	Peptic ulcer	30
Vitamin D deficiency	Isoniazid	Tuberculosis	24
	Phenobarbital	Seizure disorder	52
	Phenytoin	Seizure disorder	51
Vitamin K deficiency	Cimetidine	Peptic ulcer	29
	Moxalactam	Bronchitis; pneumonia	22
	Phenobarbital	Seizure disorder	52
	Phenytoin	Seizure disorder	51
	Quinidine	Heart disease	2
Weight gain	Amiodarone	Heart disease	3
	Chlorpromazine	Psychosis	60
	Chlorpropamid	Diabetes	39
	Diflunisal	Osteoarthritis	45
	Fenoprofen	Osteoarthritis	45
	Fluphenazine	Psychosis	61
	Guanethidine	Hypertension	9
	Ibuprofen[†]	Osteoarthritis	45
	Indomethacin	Osteoarthritis	45
	Ketoprofen	Osteoarthritis	45
	Lithium	Psychosis	58
	Meclofenamate	Osteoarthritis	45
	Minoxidil	Hypertension	8

PROBLEM	DRUG CAUSING PROBLEM	DISEASE PRESENT IF THIS DRUG IS TAKEN	PAGE
	Naproxen	Osteoarthritis	45
	Nifedipine	Hypertension	11
	Perphenazine	Psychosis	61
	Pindolol	Hypertension	10
	Piroxicam	Osteoarthritis	45
	Prazosin	Hypertension	9
	Prednisone	Asthma; rheumatoid arthritis	20,43
	Propylthiouracil	Thyrotoxicosis	41
	Rauwolfia	Hypertension	9
	Sulindac	Osteoarthritis	46
	Thioridazine	Psychosis	61
	Thiothixene	Psychosis	61
	Tolmetin	Osteoarthritis	46
Weight loss	Amphotericin B	AIDS; fungal infection	80,84
	Bisacodyl	Constipation	36
	Captopril	Hypertension	7
	Colchicine	Gout	46
	Digoxin	Heart disease	1
	Enalapril	Hypertension	8
	Methotrexate	Cancer	75
	Penicillamine	Rheumatoid arthritis	43
	Phenolphthalin	Constipation	36
	Senna	Constipation	36

*Drugs listed with warfarin as imposing risk of hemorrhage are those that increase this risk due to their anti-vitamin K effects.

†Ibuprofen is an NSAID available without prescription and can cause anemia, hyperkalemia, and weight gain.

‡Osteoporosis can be caused by other corticosteroids as well as prednisone.

Patient Information Index (Index to Appendix C)

PATIENT GROUP	PROBLEM	DRUGS AND DIETS CAUSING	PAGE
		Insulin and no food	125
		Propranolol	126
Fungal infection	Folate deficiency	Pyrimethamine	130
	Nausea, headache, vomiting	Griseofulvin and alcohol	130
		Ketoconazole	130
		Metronidazole and alcohol	130
Gout	Bleeding	Allopurinol	128
	Weight loss	Colchicine	127–128
Hypertensives	High blood sugar	Thiazides	121
	High cholesterol	Thiazides	122
	Loss of appetite	Captopril	122
	Potassium loss	Thiazides	121
	Weight gain	Minoxidil	122
Neurological	Gastritis	Levodopa	128
	Vitamin loss	Phenobarbital	128
		Phenytoin	128
Peptic ulcer	Muscle weakness	Antacids	124
Psychiatric	Weight gain	Chlorpromazine	129
		Thioridazine	129
	High blood pressure	Phenelzine and aged cheese	129
	Confusion	Lithium, diuretics, and low-salt diet	120,129
Urinary infection	Stomach irritation	Nitrofurantoin without food	131

Drug Index

V

W